Business and Health Planning for General Practice

Peter Edwards
General Practitioner, Cardiff, and Senior Research Fellow,
University of Wales College of Medicine

Stephen Jones
Service Development Manager,
Cardiff Fundholding Group

Stephanie Williams
Primary Care Facilitator,
Valleys Health Group, Honorary Lecturer
University of Wales College of Medicine

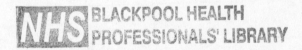

BLACKPOOL HEALTH
PROFESSIONALS' LIBRARY

Provided as an educational service by

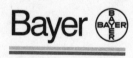

Bayer

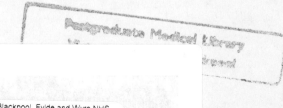

©1994 Radcliffe Medical Press Ltd, 15 Kings Meadow,
Ferry Hinksey Road, Oxford, OX2 0DP, UK

141 Fifth Avenue, New York, 10010 NY, USA

British Library Cataloguing in Publication Data

A catalogue record for this book is available from the British Library.

ISBN 1 85775 056 X

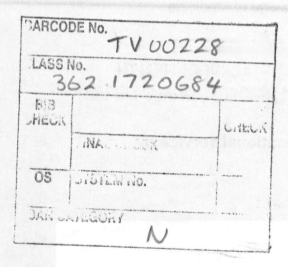
Typeset by AMA Graphics Ltd., Preston
Printed and bound in Great Britain by
T. J. Press (Padstow) Ltd., Padstow, Cornwall

Contents

Preface

This book has been written as a result of the experiences which we have accumulated both from Ely Bridge Surgery and the Department of Postgraduate Studies at the University of Wales College of Medicine.

We describe and explain the everyday problems which face those working in general practice, based upon the solutions which have been implemented in the surgery and also observed by us locally.

Many individuals have helped us. We would particularly like to acknowledge the support of our families, the partners and staff of Ely Bridge Surgery (especially Geoff Morgan for his reading of our early drafts), our colleagues at the Department of Postgraduate Studies, and all those involved in healthcare in South Wales with whom we have had contact.

Peter Edwards
Stephen Jones
Stephanie Williams

Cardiff, 1994

Introduction

General practice has much in common with other small-to-medium-sized businesses. In this context, it is perhaps instructive to consider the following extract from *A business plan* by Alan West[1].

> Management will lack skills in a number of areas. A company may be founded by an engineer who rapidly becomes faced with problems of finance, selling and promotion, which may easily lead the company into difficulties if not properly understood. The knowledge possessed by management of any of the key problems facing the company may be limited. Management will lack the time to carry out many of the complex tasks that the growing business will demand, and because of the limited financial resources will not be able to recruit the staff to handle these problems. This is a common experience of many businesses, that management spend all their time 'fire-fighting' and do not pay sufficient attention to the developmental aspects of their business.
>
> Management will react to problems rather than trying to foresee them and plan to cope with them. In common with larger organizations, the employees of the company are unlikely to be fully informed of the likely prospects for the firm, which may make rapid change of direction difficult. These are the features which characterize the small business as one which muddles along from day to day. Rather than controlling its destiny, it allows itself to be controlled.

If the above comments bring a wry smile to the face of the reader, the next extract should encourage taking the concepts of business and health planning seriously.

> . . . research in the United States on a large number of small companies shows that the stability of growth measured over 5 to 10 years is closely correlated with the amount of planning that has taken place. Short-term success does not appear to be greatly affected by the amount of planning that the business carries out, but planning is fundamental to long-term profitable survival.

The aim of this book is to develop the rationale behind the need for a strategic approach to planning in general practice, and then provide the reader with a step-by-step approach to the practical aspects of constructing a business or health plan. The comprehensive appendices give examples from the authors' own practice to illustrate the concepts discussed in the main text.

In stark terms, the choice confronting general practice is to develop a planned and measured response that anticipates the challenges of tomorrow, or to face the prospect of potentially disruptive, externally imposed solutions.

This is equally true whether the practice is fundholding or non-fundholding, and this book addresses both types of practice.

Reference

1.   West A (1988) *A business plan.* Pitman, London.

The following abbreviations are used without further explanation in the text, as they are thought to be familiar to potential readers working in primary health care.

DoH	Department of Health
FHSA	Family Health Services Authority
LMC	Local Medical Committee
NHS	National Health Service
RCGP	Royal College of General Practitioners
RHA	Regional Health Authority
SFA	Statement of Fees and Allowances

1 | A Strategic Approach to Planning for General Practice

Strategic planning is often dismissed in general practice because resources (skills, time and money) are not available, and it is considered as an activity that only very large companies can afford. This reveals a lack of awareness of its relevance to general practice. The purpose behind strategic planning is to change the management dimensions from short-term reactive to medium/long-term proactive, ie so that the practice anticipates future events rather than simply reacting to events as they happen. Strategic planning should be a continuing programme and not a one-off exercise, so that a flexible approach can be taken to changing circumstances.

The process and the benefits of strategic planning are summarized in Box 1.1. The aim of this chapter is to develop the concepts embodied in this summary from first principles, as a thorough understanding of the principles is essential to a successful planning outcome.

Why your practice needs a plan

- To achieve success.
- To avoid failure.
- To focus on the next year's activities.
- To gain commitment to goals.
- To prepare for change.

For medical practices the principles remain the same whether the issue at hand is the current and long-term financial position of the practice or the operation of fundholding within the practice. Essentially, four questions are being asked.

Box 1.1   Process and benefits of strategic planning

Strategic planning at the practice level should:

- evaluate the current strategic position
- identify all possible opportunities/threats
- identify available resources and skills
- examine the practice environment
- analyse the gap between where the practice wants to be and where it is
- develop competitive strategies for change and growth.

Benefits of a strategic plan include:

- integration and structure
- organization
- improved performance
- better use of resources
- development of new products and resources.

Benefits of the planning process include:

- teamwork and ownership
- continuous review
- learning of planning skills
- better articulation of information needs
- uprooting of dogma
- strategic understanding
- more confidence about the future.

- How did we get to where we are?
- Where do we wish to go in the future?
- How do we get there?
- What do we do to ensure it happens?

Each of these questions will be addressed in turn as this chapter unfolds.

The strategic approach for medical practices is an attempt to evaluate the present position of the business of medical practice, with reference to the business as it has evolved over previous years, its current competitors and its consumers. This cannot be done without taking note of the environment in which the business currently operates, ie the 'market'. This may simply consist of other local practices or encompass the wider NHS internal market for health care services.

The business can be reviewed in terms of the opportunities and threats that exist, both inside and outside the practice, compared to the skills and resources possessed by the business. This will allow some measure to be made of the 'gap' between where the business is and where it should be. Having done this, a strategy can be developed to minimize the shortfall. These points are illustrated in Figure 1.1, which shows the decline of a practice that has no strategic business plan, how practice goals can be set to prevent that decline, and action planned to reach the required goal.

How did we get to where we are now?

Relevant information

In order to answer this question, certain key activities are required:

- a review of the current activities and services provided by the practice; this will include as a minimum a review of the practice structure (number of partners, support and attached staff, together with an assessment of individual skills), of current practice activities (eg surgery hours, health promotion, minor surgery and non-NHS services), of the patient profile (demography and socioeconomic status) and of referral patterns (where patients are referred and why).

- an analysis of the strengths and weaknesses of the internal organization of the practice and its services, together with the opportunities and threats posed by the external environment in which the practice is operating.

Information that is useful in these processes is shown in Box 1.2.

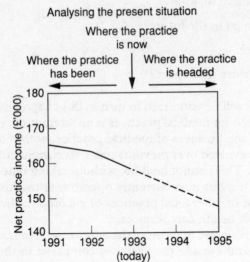

Analysing the present situation

Where the practice
is now

Where the practice
has been

Where the practice
is headed

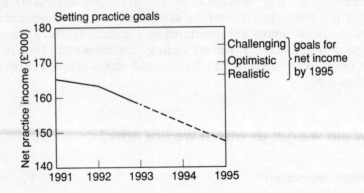

Setting practice goals

Challenging ⎫ goals for
Optimistic ⎬ net income
Realistic   ⎭ by 1995

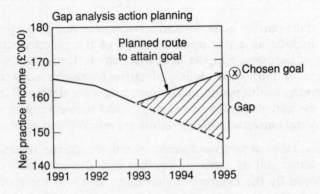

Gap analysis action planning

Planned route
to attain goal

Chosen goal

Gap

Figure 1.1   Progress of a practice with and without strategic planning.

Box 1.2   Relevant information for assessing current position

- Practice demography, trends in list size, local housing developments
- General medical service activity levels (night calls, consultation rates)
- Social factors of practice
- Population/locality
- Referral rates
- Number and type of employed/attached staff
- Profitability (compared with target)
- Comparative performance with other practices
- Impending service changes (FHSA or DoH)
- Available internal and external resources

The planning process

The process of planning should be:

- structured (with appropriate purpose, process, outcome and audit components)
- synergistic (so that the product is greater than the sum of all the components)
- participatory (as ultimate success will depend on everyone having ownership of the product).

Such a strategy will accrue the benefits of better use of resources, improved performance and integration of activities. Even greater than these are the benefits that accrue from the participants being actively involved in the *process* of planning. These include:

- improving teamwork
- ownership of outcomes
- articulation of business needs
- continuous development
- confidence in the future.

Inevitably, there are costs to such an exercise, as meaningful planning does take time.

Care must be taken to avoid the traps in planning. There may be considerable resistance to change due to participants having explicit or hidden vested interests or the group developing collective 'mind-set'. In any group of individuals, and particularly in one that has evolved over a period of time, group members accumulate emotional baggage, develop internal power structures and determine operational preferences, all of which are aimed at preserving the status quo. Vested interests are easily identified, whereas collective mind-set only becomes apparent when the group is no longer prepared to consider new ideas/alternatives or to think laterally. Clear vision and perseverance, combined with good team management, determine the route to success.

Where to start?

Evaluation of the relative business position of an organization can be achieved by a number of methods. One method commonly used is SWOT (Strengths, Weaknesses, Opportunities, Threats) analysis, which has the particular advantage of providing information in a format that is fairly rigorous, yet easy to understand. It aims to take the information gleaned and present this in a format applicable to the practice. Producing a SWOT analysis goes some way to answering the first of the four questions posed earlier.

The method is sufficiently straightforward in concept to be immediately and readily applied to general practice, as it can be used without resort to extensive information systems. SWOT analysis is highly subjective, however, in determining which practice attributes are assessed under the different categories. As none of these attributes is absolute, care must be taken to exclude bias wherever possible.

The following sections illustrate how key strengths, weaknesses, opportunities and threats could be assessed in a practice of today.

Strengths

- Experienced partnership team made up of (number) partners who bring a wide range of relevant skills to the management of the practice.

- Operating from a purpose-built surgery constructed in (date) with a full complement of ancillary and attached staff.

- High degree of commitment among the partners and staff to develop a set of shared objectives.

- Willingness on the part of the partners and staff to make use of professional management support to address recognized weaknesses in the organization.

- Open internal communications that involve all the partners in discussion on the development of the practice.

- High quality of service that is recognized by the FHSA and peers.

- High level of computerization and data recording.

Weaknesses

- Ill-defined internal organization that has resulted in confusion in the management process.

- Lack of experience in management techniques among the partners and no management-grade staff.

- Absence of formal planning and review processes.

- Consensus management and joint decision-making have inhibited action in key areas and resulted in some confusion in communications with staff, patients and external agencies.

- Inadequate management information systems for the complex task of operating fundholding.

- Lack of experience in fundholding issues and involvement in health care planning.

- Lack of effective communication of the practice vision, values and culture to all staff.

- Lack of management skills and resources to assess the efficiency, effectiveness and quality of non-clinical aspects of the practice.

- No detailed cost–benefit analyses performed for services provided and planned.

Opportunities

- The government is now offering GPs the option to hold and operate their own budgets. This development is being promoted as a means by which GPs can improve benefits to patients through improvements in operating efficiency.

- Further computerization presents an opportunity for the practice to make improvements in operational efficiency while maintaining or improving standards of service.

- By embracing modern management techniques and developing internal management skills, the partners should be able to achieve improvements in working conditions.

Threats

- The pressure of patient demand is expected to increase, as a result of both the promotion of new services under the new contract for GPs and an ageing patient population.

- The increasing demands for the partners to become involved in the management of the practice could ultimately lead to a reduction in the standards of patient care and/or increase time pressures on the partners.

- The introduction of fundholding may start a trend towards a two-tier GP service. The decision to accept/reject fundholding for emotional reasons alone could disadvantage the practice/patients in the medium term.

SWOT – so what?

It is important that strengths and weaknesses are evaluated from an external perspective, ie from the point of view of someone outside the practice. Too often an internal perspective generates what are known as 'motherhood' statements, eg 'high-quality care' and 'an established practice'. A practice attribute is only a strength if it is perceived as such by an external party, eg the patient.

This external perspective is very important to the use of SWOT analysis, as there is a critical distinction between what the partners think is important in the practice and what the patient considers important. However difficult the partners may sometimes find patients (or other external parties) to be, it is they who ultimately 'consume' the service.

It is likely that a practice will have more items in each SWOT category than in the example above. Quite often it is difficult to decide in which category (or categories) a practice attribute should be placed. For example, the retirement of a partner may provide the opportunity for change, growth and development, while it poses a threat from the departure of an experienced team member and the need to find a replacement. From the list of entries in each of the SWOT categories, it is possible to develop an action strategy. In essence, these strategies should be to:

- effectively match strengths to opportunities

- convert (or neutralize) weaknesses and threats

- enhance creativity and develop innovation.

This is achieved in practice by a process of action planning, ie breaking down the strategy into a series of measurable, manageable and distributable steps, and implementation.

Opportunities and threats need to be assessed in terms of both the likelihood of their actually happening (probability) and their significance to the practice if they do happen (impact). Each item recorded as an opportunity or threat can be scored on a scale of 0–10 for both probability and impact. It is then possible to plot these variables separately for opportunities and threats, as shown in Figure 1.2. Items that are located in the 'red zone' require urgent response by the practice as they are very likely to happen and will have a significant effect when they do. The practice must have a response strategy ready to deal with these factors. 'Green zone' items are less immediate and can be dealt with over a longer time frame. The 'amber zone' factors are more difficult to assess, as they could move in either direction over a period of time. It can be seen, however, that an item with medium probability and low impact can be compared with one of medium probability and high impact, and implications drawn.

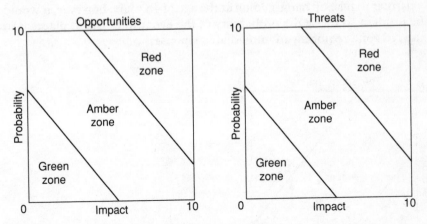

Figure 1.2 Assessment of the probability and impact of opportunities and threats.

As an example, consider the plotting of two possibilities in a three-partner practice: a new development of 300 houses inside the practice area and one of the partners being on long-term sick leave. The housing development, plotted as an opportunity, would have a moderate impact (5) due to list size effects but a low probability (2) as planning permission has only just been granted. In this planning year, the event thus falls into the amber zone close to the green; however, a re-evaluation next year may show no change in impact, but a change in probability (to 8) as the building starts. This now becomes an amber item approaching red and requires more attention.

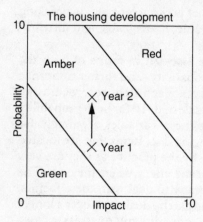

Figure 1.3   Assessment of the probability and impact of the housing development.

The partners in the practice may be fit and well, so while the prolonged absence of one would have have a high impact as a threat (9) due to the extra workload, there is no reason to suspect anything other than a low probability (2), which places such an event safely in the amber zone. Were a partner to take up hang-gliding at the age of 46 years, however, it would be prudent to revise the probability of the event to 6, which places it in the red zone requiring an immediate response.

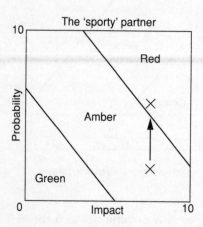

Figure 1.4   Assessment of the probability and impact of the 'sporty' partner.

Importantly, when this exercise is repeated annually, it is possible to measure the impact of the practice response strategy; for example, has item X now moved from the red zone to the amber zone or vice versa? It also allows both new and redundant opportunities and threats to be added to or removed from the plot as appropriate.

A proforma SWOT analysis and opportunities/threats matrices for individual completion are included in Appendix A.

Where do we wish to go in the future?

The mission statement

The analysis of why the practice needs a strategic plan has so far determined the present position of the practice in relation to its external environment and has also reviewed how it arrived there. The second item to determine is where the practice wishes to go, and this can often be summarized by a statement of values, which is often referred to as a *mission statement*. This is a statement of purpose for the practice, which enumerates:

* who the practice (team) is
* the boundaries to the practice (in both activity and geography)
* the `business' of the practice
* how the business will be conducted
* the standards that apply.

The purpose of the mission statement is shown in Box 1.3. The mission statement should be the driving force of the practice, and all activity undertaken should be directed towards the achievement of the mission. SWOT analysis is a valuable aid in converting implicit assumptions about hopes, aspirations, fears and motivations into explicit statements that can be focused into a mission statement.

The process of producing the mission statement is at least as important as final agreed statement itself. The more focused the mission statement, the easier it will be to identify the practice objectives. To this end, the mission statement needs to be:

* roughly right
* enduring
* succinct

Box 1.3   Purpose of a mission statement in the planning process

* To provide a common thread
* To motivate employees
* To act as a focus for policies and objectives
* To provide a global framework for planning

- memorable
- believable
- energizing to all concerned with it[1].

The potential benefits of a good, workable, mission statement are:

- the key values of the practice are made explicit
- a strategic framework for practice planning is created
- motivation factors are incorporated into practice goals.

The factors associated with the creation of an unusable mission statement include the incorporation of unmeasurable qualities or unrealistic expectations, and failure to involve and communicate with all the team members, thereby being divisive.

Practice objectives

Having decided on the basic philosophy of the practice and its relative position, it is necessary to determine:

- where the practice is actually heading
- if this is not the destination sought, how the desired goal can be achieved by changing the strategic direction of the practice.

In other words, the mission statement has to be underpinned by a series of practice objectives to achieve the mission. These should incorporate:

- formal statement of vision, objectives and priorities
- agreed structure, roles and responsibilities
- statement of working profile (how, when, where)
- support systems required
- support staffing required
- resource implications.

Typical practice objectives identified (but not quantified or prioritized at this stage) as part of the outline business planning exercise could include:

- the need to provide the optimal level of patient care within the partnership and within available resources

- development of shared objectives from individual agendas and incorporation into the practice vision and strategy

- expressing the acceptable balance between the business and vocation of general practice

- optimizing the balance of personal and practice time, bearing in mind the effect on resources and objectives, particularly for non-core activities, eg acting as a factory medical officer, which will have effects on total practice income

- accepting the need for delegation of the management function.

These objectives should be discussed openly and specific agreement reached on each. For some objectives differences in opinion might only be accommodated by not taking a formal or definitive stance, and the tolerance of the practice as a whole must be decided in such instances.

Option appraisal

Practice objectives now need:

- prioritization where there are specific resource implications (most will fall into this category, even demands on particularly valuable but uncosted partnership time)

- time for individual reflection and structured, collective discussion to ensure that outcomes are reached without sacrificing any participation or team goodwill.

The next step is therefore to make some assessment of priority. *Option appraisal* is an aid to decision-making when allocating resources, as deciding where the practice wants to go will inevitably require a review of the resources available to get there. It assists by improving the quality and relevance of information supplied to the decision-making process, so that the final decision is based on rational, consistent criteria.

Option appraisal is based on the notion of scarcity of resources. Where there is competition for resources, the criterion of choice should be efficiency of resource consumption. There are two components of assessment:

- cost–benefit analysis, which attempts to resolve which options are viable and desirable

- cost–effectiveness analysis, which examines how the resources should be utilized.

It must be stressed that option appraisal is not a substitute for managerial judgement. Its use, however, does permit all relevant data on the various options to be considered in a consistent format. The availability of all relevant material pertinent to the decision is a significant aid to the efficient allocation of resources.

The major benefits of option appraisal are as follows.

- It is a disciplined approach that ensures that all relevant factors are considered in an explicit and systematic manner.
- It provides an opportunity to ensure that all valid alternative ways of meeting the objectives are considered.
- It is an effective means of marshalling the arguments for and against particular solutions.
- It is a recognized mechanism for obtaining the endorsement of those with authority to approve major expenditure.
- It acts as the basis for detailed planning, thus ensuring that policy can be followed through into detailed activity.

The major disadvantage of option appraisal is that it takes time, consuming a considerable amount of management and planning resources. Major issues deserve considerable attention, however, and when properly performed the process ensures effective use of resources and wiser decision-making. It is also important to realize that many managers approach option appraisal cynically, convinced that the outcome will merely be formalization of a decision already made. It is therefore fundamental that the constraints are quite clearly defined, and results should not be discarded for political motives.

Box 1.4 outlines the process of option appraisal in sequence, though in reality the stages may become blurred. Information obtained at a later stage may lead to a reassessment of action taken at an earlier stage. A flexible approach is therefore necessary to ensure that the most effective outcome is achieved.

Option appraisal has diverse potential applications in health care, for example:

- strategic planning – determining the relative priority to be accorded to the needs of different client groups
- service delivery – describing the full implications of policy choices and identifying those that represent the best value for money
- capital investment – particularly important because of the comparative irreversibility of choice for both buildings and equipment.

Box 1.4 Process of option appraisal

1 Define the issue/problem in the broadest terms, eg the practice appointments system is inefficient.

2 State the objectives, constraints and performance criteria. Consider
   (i) what and how much can be done to resolve the problem
   (ii) what is the least-cost way of improving matters by a given amount
   (iii) what is the most effective way to spend a given amount of resource to improve the situation.

3 Formulate possible options and reduce to a manageable number.

For an appointment system there are several options in respect of solutions. One of these is to do nothing – the 'no change' option – which permits the calculation of a benchmark by which the additional cost of gaining the extra benefit of doing *something* about the problem can be measured. In other words, if nothing is done the problem as it exists can be measured and current costs (time, money, stress etc) can be assigned. The costs associated with each of the options can then be assessed against this benchmark, rather than against zero cost.

4 Evaluate the derived options by:
   (i) detailed description
   (ii) assessment of benefits
   (iii) assessment of recurring costs
   (iv) assessment of one-off costs.

The advantages of including non-monetary values (time, stress, reputation etc) of costs and benefits into each option include:

- exploring areas of possible disagreement that are not limited to financial resources

- clarifying their magnitude in terms of personal values

- indicating whether they are significant in relation to financial costs and benefits

5 Select the preferred option from presented results.

In conclusion, option appraisal is an effective method of ensuring the systematic examination of alternative ways of meeting objectives before resources are committed. In this way, the practice gains:

- an explicit understanding of the issue to be addressed and the specific objectives to be pursued
- a full appreciation of the relative advantages and disadvantages of the alternative solutions
- identification of the option that in the *collective judgement of the practice* represents the best value for money.

How do we get there?

Putting strategic vision into operation

Having determined the preferred destination of the practice, some thought needs to be given to how to get there. Planning can be thought of as a group of interrelated activities, which together act as a series of keys that can unlock the door to success for the practice business.

The focus of strategic planning should be on the changing world within which general practice exists. The ability to accept change as the norm and to create and implement a strategic plan involves the practice in changing from reactive to proactive planning. The most attractive scenario is one in which:

- possible changes are anticipated
- the effects on the practice are calculated
- a plan is formulated to cope in a positive manner with the change.

The first stage is to draw a baseline, which allows a realistic appraisal to be made rather than striving hopelessly for a utopian ideal. It is important to come to terms with reality and start improving the business from there. A 'map' of the practice world needs to be drawn, and within this framework, current activities and workloads can be defined and then quantified. Conversion of activity and workload into monetary values can be achieved by reference to the SFA (Red Book)[2] or financial journals, but it is more difficult to analyse the context in which the work takes place. Context consists of two variables:

- those that are within the control of the practice
- those that are largely outside the control of the practice.

Some examples of the different types of factors are given in Box 1.5. The objectives for the practice must be to:

- maximize the effects of controllable factors
- minimize the effects of uncontrollable factors.

Developments in general practice can be achieved in two ways. The first is by quantum leaps, which include computerization of the practice, building or moving to new premises, introducing a practice manager, or becoming a fundholder. Secondly, development can be achieved in incremental stages, eg by developing a systematic approach to the management of change:

- determining the items that should be done as opposed to those that the practice team would like to do
- the establishment of a responsive claims system to the FHSA to ensure good cash flow management
- the introduction of monitoring systems to identify trends and exceptions in performance
- routinely reviewing planned compared with actual activity/income/ expenditure to analyse discrepancies
- the construction of an interactive information system to enhance effective decision-making within the practice.

Box 1.5 Factors governing the context in which practice work takes place

Controllable factors

- Activity mix
- Range, experience and type of staff
- Consulting arrangements
- Distribution of workload among partners

Uncontrollable factors

- Terms of service requirements
- Health and safety requirements
- Employment legislation
- FHSA policies on cash-limited expenditure
  - cost-rent schemes
  - practice staff reimbursement
  - staff training expenses

Such developments can be achieved by using planning principles to convert inputs to outputs (*see* Box 1.6) to achieve an outcome or goal.

Managing the journey

The practice may have to follow several routes if it wishes to reach its destination. It is unlikely that it will arrive safely unless the journey is carefully managed. This involves the provision of resources (money, manpower, time, space), together with a review/feedback mechanism so that deviations from course can be quickly spotted and corrected.

Any change is threatening, but mutual support and understanding go a considerable way to diminishing the threat. Moreover, many team members will need appropriate training/development to manage the transition. Identification of individual strengths and weaknesses allows tasks to be more effectively delegated while maintaining self-confidence. To maintain the timetable for change, a careful balance needs to be struck between encouraging creativity and good time management.

Within any business key people can be identified who possess the appropriate skills for the practice to function efficiently; they are required for the continued health of the business. The skills that are required by the business will require continual upgrading to meet the challenges and opportunities that arise with increasing regularity.

Many GPs have quite successfully built their practices up without the assistance of a professional manager. As the practice grows, however, a critical size is reached when no one GP can manage every aspect of the practice; at this point communication arrangements begin to fail. This poses a dilemma as to the possibilities for further growth, which will be unique to each practice due to its own characteristics and circumstances. The plaintive cry is often heard that although having a manager may be the most effective way to run the practice, the senior partner does not want to 'let go of the reins'.

Box 1.6   Inputs and outputs relevant to achieving practice goals

Inputs	**Outputs**
• Uncontrollable factors	• Improved patient services
• GPs' time	• Better use of resources
• Clinical preference	• Improved teamwork/morale
• Staff expertise	• Greater satisfaction
• Resource availability	• Enhanced remuneration

The practical issues of recruiting a practice manager are dealt with elsewhere[3], and only the general implications of such an option are considered here. A practice manager should allow the GPs, as the owners of the business, to take a strategic view of their practice. Basically, strategic vision is about the GP making a cultural leap from the *management* to the *governance* of the practice. In doing so, the nature of the role of the GP will change. The nature of issues will become more abstract and judgmental, as the GP's place on the decision-making continuum shifts from operational to strategic. The distinction between these two types of function are shown in Box 1.7.

The GP as strategist finds himself faced with difficult and complex managerial/organizational issues, which are often an uncomfortable 'fit' with clinical practice. There is often a problem of understanding the strategy process and deciding on what basis to make choices. The availability of professional management in the practice can introduce:

- analytical skills

- status/credibility

- a holistic view

- integration/key values

- control, centralized coordination and communication, thus freeing the GP to contemplate implementation and mission

- political skills

- change skills

- coaching (leadership)

- risk-taking

- decentralization (freedom within fixed parameters).

Box 1.7 Characteristics of operational and strategic issues in managerial decisions

Operational issues	Strategic decisions
• Routine	• Non-routine
• Closed decisions	• Open systems
• Good data/information available	• Require conceptualization
• Short-term/urgent issues	• Little or no hard data
	• Long-term view

It should be remembered that appointing a practice manager is concerned with giving operational freedom to others while retaining overall strategic control.

Strategic vision is currently a fashionable concept and strives to be holistic, examining every aspect of the practice. It is high level, often ambiguous and usually long term. It is certainly important. Strategic decisions are made complex by, and are fraught with, uncertainty, but remain a key focus for management. They attempt to correlate practice strategy with organizational realities in the light of incremental change, the power and politics of the partnership and the organizational culture.

What do we do to ensure it happens?

Practical considerations

The final question relates to mechanisms that ensure that the desired outcomes are delivered. Is planning the answer? Negative responses include:

- we never needed it before, so why now?
- it takes too much time and discourages initiative
- plans are inflexible, inaccurate and nobody uses them anyway
- planning is a meaningless ritual.

What should practices expect from planning? A 'good plan' will consider the radical and innovative options, allow the unthinkable to be thought and challenge the status quo and inertia of the practice. It should be neither ad hoc nor piecemeal. The planning process must engender team spirit and 'ownership' for the plan and must therefore match expectation with action.

It is easy to spend too much time analysing what has gone wrong in the past, gathering information rather than using it to make decisions. It can be difficult to focus beyond the short term, and an incrementalist or 'muddling through' approach is accepted. There are often too many vested interests and the organizational 'mindset' prohibits unconventional thinking. Practice culture may be exceptionally resistant to change, thus making ownership and commitment difficult to gain. Ultimately, deploying insufficient resources to the planning activity will ensure there is no implementation.

Communication is crucial to effective planning. Unless everyone understands the practice strategy and has ownership of the plan, individual innovative energies will be dissipated and enthusiasm deflated. Those not committed to the plan divert resources, create delay by obstructions and undermine its credibility. It is possible to gain commitment to strategic planning through:

- education/communication
- participation
- support
- negotiation
- manipulation
- coercion.

These are developed further in Chapter 2.

It must be remembered that not every eventuality envisaged in the practice plan will happen. Simply knowing that what is actually happening is different from what was predicted, however, identifies changed circumstances and thus allows the practice to respond quickly – with a revised version of the plan!

References

1. Peters TH and Waterman RH (1992) *In search of excellence.* Harper and Row, London.

2. Department of Health *National Health Service general medical services, statement of fees and allowances payable to general medical practitioners in England and Wales from 1 April 1990.* DoH, London.

3. Irvine S and Haman H (1993) *Making sense of personnel management.* Radcliffe Medical Press, Oxford.

2 | Action Planning and the Management of Change

Business planning in general practice is a means to an end, rather than an end in itself. It is a set of tools that will enable a practice to make the best use of its resources. Properly used, it can help a practice to identify how those resources (staff, premises, income, time, information) are currently being deployed and point to ways in which some or all of them might be organized more efficiently and effectively.

This inevitably implies that changes will be made. As change is an uncomfortable state of affairs for most people, this is often the point in the process at which good ideas and intentions, which sounded fine in discussions or on paper, begin to founder. Converting theory into reality is clearly crucial if any progress is to be made. The steps outlined in Box 2.1 constitute a pragmatic approach, which allows progress to be made in an incremental fashion.

Recognizing that change is necessary

The first step in managing any change effectively is to secure agreement among the practice team that a change away from present practice is needed at all. This sounds straightforward in principle, but in reality it is not. For example, it may be perfectly plain to one of the practice partners that more effort needs to be devoted to increasing the percentage of children currently being immunized. In informal discussions the practice nurse and another partner may share that view, and when the topic is raised at a practice meeting there may be general nods of agreement. This verbal or surface level assent, however, must be written into the overall practice strategy, and then needs to be translated into operational guidelines and turned into everyday activity.

Clearly, good administrative systems will be needed to reinforce any decisions to change practice activity. These include:

Box 2.1   Steps in the successful management of change

- Recognizing that change is necessary
- Gaining commitment from all involved
- Getting the authority to act
- Drawing up a plan
- Making it happen
- Evaluation of progress

- taking minutes of meetings
- following up agenda points with action
- circulating minutes in advance of meetings so that participants are reminded of their own commitments
- delegating responsibility for areas of management.

None of these administrative tasks, however, can substitute for the management task involved in effecting change.

The first management task is to define the end-point at which the practice is aiming. This is obviously one function of the business planning process itself. The more members of the team who are involved in this part of the process, the easier it will be to convince them of the merits of the operational aspects of proposed changes. Involvement in the early stages helps the practice team members to feel a sense of ownership over and commitment to the strategy.

Having determined the strategic destination, the next requirement is to plan the route by which it will be reached. It is at this point that resistance to any proposals may first be met, because it is now that staff first begin to realize that the proposed change may affect the way they do their own work. To continue the example mentioned above, everyone in the practice has agreed that the uptake of immunization needs improving. What they did not necessarily agree at the time it was discussed was the impact on other practice activity in general, and on their own activity in particular. The management task at this stage then becomes one of persuading the rest of the staff that the proposed change is a necessary one.

This stage is one of fact-finding and gathering information. The aim is to mount a convincing case for shifting resources, eg away from acute work and into a health promotion activity. Information needs to be sought on the potential benefits of this change for the practice as a whole, such as:

- an increased income for the practice
- a better standard of care for more patients.

This information can come from a variety of sources, including:

- academic departments of general practice
- standards set by local consultants
- the RCGP
- patient groups.

Information also needs to be gathered as to how the change might benefit individual members of the team, eg in the form of training, personal development opportunities, or potential publications. Similarly, information is required about any costs that may be incurred by adopting the new change. Such information encompasses the following:

- Will additional computer hardware or software be needed?
- Are any training needs immediately obvious?
- Will additional staff be required, and if so, how many and for how long?
- Equally important, what are the costs of *not* adopting the proposed change?

Involving staff in such discussions, even at this early stage, is a good tactic. It enriches the information search by increasing the type and number of sources available. It also helps to ensure that the information gathered is relevant to the practice's needs.

Gaining the commitment of those involved

Information in most organizations tends to follow gravity, flowing from the top downwards. Opening up channels so that information moves freely from the ground upwards is good practice. It will help to ensure that the policies framed are practical and relevant. It will also prepare the ground for the next stage of the process of managing change: gaining the commitment of those involved. This stage involves turning intellectual appreciation into 'gut level' commitment.

At this point, it is important to try to clarify the reasons behind the proposed change, looking critically at the objectives, and the degree of necessity involved. It is likely that the change envisaged lies somewhere along a continuum between desirable and necessary, but it is important to be clear about precisely where on the continuum the proposed change lies and to be sure that all the members of the practice are helped to see it in the same terms. Fitting the proposed change into the practice's overall aims is a good way of helping the whole team to appreciate its significance.

This is particularly difficult, and correspondingly important, in the case of attached staff with different objectives set by other authorities. For example, the practice may wish that the attached health visitor would do more work with the elderly and be keen to involve her in surveillance of the over 75s. The health visitor's nurse manager, however, may be less keen to reduce the health visitor's caseload of under 5s. The practice manager in this situation must do some careful preparatory work to find out exactly what constraints operate on the health visitor's time and what scope there is for releasing time from her work with the under 5s. The manager also needs to know something about the health visitor's present skills and aspirations.

- Does she need to brush up on her assessments of the elderly?

- Does she fully understand the new procedures and changes in the process of referring patients for social care, which came into being with the Community Care Act 1993?

- Does she need more training? If so, will the practice pay for it? If the nurse manager does not enthusiastically support the proposed change in her health visitor's work, it is unlikely that the community unit will fund any additional training.

- What are the health visitor's longer term career hopes and ambitions, as these may affect her willingness or reluctance to undertake new work with the over 75s?

The purpose of all this fact-finding is to increase knowledge of what motivates the health visitor and the constraints under which she works, to be in a better position to accurately anticipate the impact of any proposed change on her daily activity. Anticipating possible objections will help in planning an effective strategy to overcome them.

Similar principles apply to the other staff. Faced with proposals that affect the way they do their work, they may react in a variety of ways. One of the most common reactions is fear. Some people welcome change as an opportunity, which indeed it is, but many also fear change, not least because it implies that they may have to meet new standards, which may or may not be clear at the outset. This in turn raises the fear that they may fail and will consequently be made to look incompetent. Although this point may seem self-evident it is worth stressing, because an individual's sense of self-worth is closely linked to performance at work and such fears are very common. Recognizing that these fears exist among most staff is a necessary first step to defusing their impact.

Techniques for overcoming resistance

The ways of gaining commitment to strategic planning have already been listed (*see* page 21). They are extended here as specific techniques for overcoming resistance to change.

- Demonstration: studies of effective change management in medical contexts indicate that using practical demonstrations of how a proposed change will work, or is working in another practice, is an effective technique in overcoming resistance to change.

- Support: the individual members of staff who will be most strongly affected by a proposed change may need additional support to help them to cope with the inevitable disruptions to their routine working patterns.

- Mapping key relationships: identifying prevailing patterns of influence in different working groups within the practice is a good way to target opinion leaders. Drawing these individuals into devising ways to implement changes at an early stage in the planning process decreases the number of potential sources of resistance and increases commitment to the plans themselves. *Force field analysis:* this can be a useful tool for illustrating the forces for and against new proposals, as shown in Box 2.2. Taking force field analysis into account will help to prepare effectively for any anticipated opposition.

- Negotiation: in some circumstances it may be appropriate to adjust the nature or degree of the proposed change to meet the interests of potentially resistant individuals, particularly if such resistance will lead to impasse. Although this negotiation may slow the pace of change, it will at least keep change going forward.

- Manipulation: this approach is a deliberate attempt to sidestep resistance rather than to tackle it head-on. It involves the selective dissemination of information, and as such is a 'buy now, pay later' tactic.

- Coercion: when all else fails, and all prospects of reaching a consensus have evaporated, the senior partner can pull rank. This tactic might involve either implicit or explicit threats of loss of promotion or future prospects, or break-up of the partnership. It is unwise to use this tactic unless any threats made can/will be carried out.

These approaches can be used singly or in combination, depending on the likely reactions involved in the process of change. They should be employed sensitively and constructively, bearing in mind the long-term implications of solving the immediate problem of turning resistance to change into positive commitment to the proposed change.

Getting the authority to act

This stage involves the formal or informal transfer of authority to implement the proposed change. It makes sense, in both operational and strategic terms, to formalize this transfer. Delegating such authority provides a focal point for contributions of ideas and energies (and complaints). It also helps to avoid the 'nobody's job' syndrome where tasks are ignored because everyone thought someone else was responsible for them, when in fact nobody was.

In deciding how authority should be delegated, it is helpful to analyse how a proposed change is going to affect each member of the team, both in relation to the work each currently does and in relation to the new work. Anticipating the difficulties that staff are likely to meet in trying to implement new changes will help in planning ways of avoiding those difficulties.

Key relationships should be mapped out to see how they will be affected by new working patterns. It can be useful to identify who will 'gain' and who is likely to 'lose' from the proposed change, as well as who the decision-makers will be and who controls access to crucial information in the current situation.

Good communication is important at this stage, so that people are kept informed of developments.

Box 2.2 Force field analysis in the management of change

Forces in favour	Forces against
• Better quality of care	• Time away from present tasks
• Better service to patients	• More demands from patients
• Better understanding of the process	• More new tasks for staff
• Opportunities for practice-based learning	• Need for more training

Managing change – implementing plans

This stage provides the opportunity to avoid the whole process of change falling at the first hurdle. Involving the staff most affected by the proposed change will ensure that the plans devised will work and that the staff will be happy to implement them. The converse is equally true.

- Process: flow charts can be used to map out the intended new process and pinpoint ways in which it will differ from the existing process. The thinking behind the change should be explained to the staff and their objections heard – they are likely to be acutely aware of operational (practical) constraints, so their suggestions will make sense.

  This will help to ensure that the present position in relation to the proposed change is clear to all practice staff, which will in turn assist in drawing up appropriate performance indicators, so that progress towards the intended destination can be measured.

- Costs: any estimates/guesstimates should now be turned into quotations, the accuracy of costings should be checked and the sources of payment should be accurately identified.

- Training: existing skills should be matched to new tasks at this point and any training needs identified.

Making change happen successfully

This step involves managing the journey from plan to destination. One of the key steps at this stage is phasing the implementation of the change. The potential for costly mistakes is decreased when major changes to systems are introduced in a stepwise rather than a wholesale fashion. Similarly, if an early 'pay-off' for staff can be built into the process, this will help to improve motivation to continue to implement, rather than to sabotage, a new system.

Delegation of responsibility for implementing specific tasks or processes is another good motivational technique. Sharing responsibility for the success of the new process will also help to generate commitment to it.

Finally, building an evaluation framework and a time-scale for review into the change process will help to ensure that all staff are kept informed of early successes and have the opportunity to learn from any mistakes. Such an approach will foster an atmosphere of constructive debate, which is essential to any team hoping to improve the quality of its output.

3 | Information for Planning

Planning requires information. Present trends in the NHS make collecting information that is relevant to planning and managing services a difficult task. This is because until now much effort has been focused on information technology at the expense of information use. Momentum towards collecting information is currently increasing, however, to which the following factors contribute:

- pressure for accountability within the NHS
- emphasis on a general management function within the NHS
- emphasis on efficient use of scarce resources
- changes in NHS structures so that decision-making is being devolved to smaller units.

Medical records in planning

The definition of 'record' is 'to register in permanent form'. The medical record is, therefore, a permanent list of the health events that occur to each patient, and a clinically based data collection process is proposed as the key to future health planning. This will be achieved by incorporating 'health event linkages' into the process, so that a complete picture emerges.

What is recorded?

Demographic information is recorded in order to identify each individual patient. Characteristically, this consists of name, address and date of birth. Each patient has an NHS number, which is no longer unique, although there are plans for a new numbering system to be issued in the future. Any referral made through a computer system in a fundholding practice has an identifying number. Within computerized practices each patient also has a number. With the practice code number, these three numbers create a unique identifier for a health event for each patient.

The clinical information relating to a patient episode/event can be recorded in a variety of ways, which will allow different degrees of accessibility. Within the clinical record it is likely that the date of each consultation will be recorded, together with some or all of the following (not necessarily in this order):

- symptoms offered by the patient
- examination(s) made
- investigation ordered, with subsequent results
- diagnosis made
- prescription given
- comments
- health promotion data.

The assembly of the component parts is no different whatever *type* of technology used, be that Lloyd George envelopes, A4 folders or computer systems. The retrieval of the data, and therefore the amount of information that is available about each individual patient and also about the practice population, varies depending on the *structure* of the record. Enthusiasts of each type of recording method will say that if used properly, it will allow a picture to be built up for each patient by using summaries, and for the practice by using registers and manual or computerized databases.

One major impact of a computer system is that if used to record each diagnosis (health event) for each patient, the amount and value of information that is readily available will be increased dramatically. Analysis of this perceived morbidity is vital for the planning of future health care services.

Information needs of primary care

Information needs within the NHS today mean that a fresh approach must be taken to collection, storage, retrieval and reporting of information in the community setting. It is no longer appropriate for isolated parties to look only at their own part of the jigsaw. A more complete picture of the care provided for patients in the community is required.

Unfortunately, the variety of information collection systems currently in use in the NHS make this difficult. Developing an information strategy for the practice that allows a complete picture of care for all groups to be drawn, however, is of great benefit to the practice – information is power.

The only logical answer within primary care is to devise a system based on individual patient data as the building block, and then to look at ways of facilitating appropriate sharing of information. This is the only way, for example, that a community services provider will be able to provide accurate information for a GP fundholder contract. An integrated patient information system is required to give a complete picture of patient contacts with health professionals.

Patient information systems should enable patient-based information to be aggregated to a level at which it can fulfil a number of requirements. Although the system should be first and foremost a tool for health professionals to enhance the care they give to patients, the following information needs should also be met as by-products of such an operational patient management system.

- Contracts: activity and performance information relating to contracts that the health authority and GP fundholders have with the community services provider is required by the FHSA to facilitate GP fundholding and the planning of primary health care services.

- Audit: comprehensive patient-based morbidity and dependency data will facilitate medical and clinical audit. Information may also be required for research purposes.

- Management: better information is required on which to plan services, make decisions for both investment and disinvestment in services/facilities and therefore manage the services in order to provide better value for money.

- Health needs: health needs assessment is another crucial area in which there is currently a lack of even baseline information about morbidity and associated dependency to inform decision making.

- Sharing: underpinning all of the above is the need to share information in order to eliminate waste of resources in gathering data and ensure that a complete picture of patient care is compiled. It is then necessary to aggregate such data so that locality/district needs can also be identified.

Information for the annual report

A clearly specified amount of information is required to be submitted as an annual report to the FHSA. Some of this information is simple and straightforward to collect. With a little extra effort and planning, this information collection process can be made to work for the practice. The information that is collected can improve the capacity of the practice to monitor progress towards the objectives that have been outlined in the business plan.

The audit process is applied in order to check the extent to which the practice complies with the requirements of the annual report. All the information outined in Box 3.1 can be thought of as 'mandatory audit', in the sense that the information is required under the *Terms of service for doctors in general practice*, colloquially known as the Contract (1990), for the annual report. Although the information required represents the essential minimum, the systems needed to achieve adequate audit in these areas can be applied in a far wider context.

Detailed information is given in Appendix B.

Attitudes to computerization

Modern general practice requires GPs to consider extending their range of computerization due to the considerable information handling necessary for effective management of the clinical, business and (possibly) fundholding aspects of the practice. Many GPs have become more content to have computers in their practices, but fundholding may be the stimulus for bringing a terminal into the consulting room. This option needs careful assessment and sensitive handling, as there are many reasons why GPs and other staff are apprehensive about (further) computerizing their practice, some of which are considered below.

There is a fear of redundancy of both the job and the job-holder's skills. Although objective experience shows that the actual number of jobs seldom declines, the nature of the jobs may change considerably. This is equally applicable to clinical and non-clinical staff. Inevitably, there will

---

Box 3.1   Information to be provided in the annual report

- Staff
- Premises
- Referrals
- External commitments
- Patient comments
- Prescribing

be concern that those using the computer terminals will damage them (repair costs can be considerable), which often manifests itself as not understanding the computer – or not wanting to!

Many GPs believe that having a terminal on the desk changes the GP/patient relationship; however, there is no evidence that such a change is necessarily detrimental to patient care. Were this so, the drive by GPs themselves for computers would long since have faltered. GPs point to changes in eye contact with patients as one of the major differences that arises from having a terminal in the consulting room, but they also acknowledge that deficiencies in skills with the new system, particularly keyboard skills, will mean that consulting in the new environment will consume extra time initially. Those who are not advocates of computerization often fear the danger of 'expert syndrome' being created in the partnership, and the plaintive cry of: 'How does it help me? I'm a doctor not a computer operator,' is heard at this point.

None of these issues is insurmountable, provided that the reasons for the changes are adequately explained to the concerned individual.

Information technology requirements

Irrespective of whether a practice already has a computer, the introduction of information technology into the practice, particularly if it is fundholding, will require a thorough review of current practice capabilities. Some relevant considerations have been included in Appendix C.

Data capture

The collection of data by current systems, either manual or by computer, has proved to be woefully inadequate. This situation could be improved by the introduction of a system of bar codes and hand-held light pens for use by appropriate community professional staff, eg district nurses and health visitors. This method of data capture lends itself readily to the type of services provided in the wide variety of locations in the community including patients' own homes. The advantages of using light pens/bar codes include:

- the system is quick to use

- it is very accurate

- validation checks are built in

- little training is required

- it is relatively inexpensive in comparison with other forms of data collection, eg laptop computers, within the community.

The introduction of a community operational support system should enhance multidisciplinary working and improve commissioning and contracting information. This should allow the development of integrated care, outcome measures and more effective management of resources (including the identification of costs). The issue of developing localized accountability and responsibility can also be explored. The objectives of introducing such a system would be:

- to give the health team access to a patient-based information system, to enable it to plan and manage its own workloads, meet agreed performance targets and undertake clinical audit, which would enhance team work and thereby improve patient care

- to generate improved information for assessment of health needs, health gain investment decisions and planning of service developments, particularly in support of providing a wider range of services in the community rather than in hospital

- to reduce costs through the integration of systems

- improve data quality and the speed of information flow.

The type of information that should be recorded is shown in Box 3.2. Management information can also be recorded, for example:

- the length of time spent by staff in meetings

- the number of health promotion sessions

- recorded mileage

- travelling time.

Once this area comes under discussion, even more radical innovations become apparent. As an example, it would be possible to record whether a patient is medically housebound (does not leave the house for any reason) or merely socially housebound (where lack of transport is the major reason for needing care and attention at home). If this second category were found to be a significant proportion of the population, particularly among the elderly, it might be worthwhile copying the example of the supermarkets and providing free transport (to the surgery) so that care could be given there.

The information could also be used to prepare a management plan, in which all members of the team treating a patient could record their contribution/view on the plan of action. The patient should also be able to contribute, particularly in chronic or palliative care situations. At some

---

Box 3.2 Data items collected in a community operational support system

- Name
- Sex
- Date of birth
- Address
- Name of GP
- Contract number
- Health or social care worker
- Date of first contact
- First contact/repeat visit
- Diagnosis
- Dependency
- Type of intervention
- Length of intervention
- Location of intervention
- Referral details
- Outcome

---

point in the future it might also be possible to devise a system based on bar codes that would allow patients the opportunity to record their views on the quality of service that they receive from the different professional groups who serve them. This would certainly be a move away from traditional consumer surveys and might provide more accurate and timely information.

Information interchange/management

Activity information systems, in both general practice and hospitals, are now widely used to create performance indicators and to facilitate medical audit. Furthermore, in the new NHS internal market, they form the basis for financial information, billing and resource allocation.

Such an approach, which introduces a case-mix dimension to management issues, has a number of advantages.

- It uses readily available patient data.

- It categorizes/identifies patients with similar resource expectations.

- The development of 'standard case' definitions allows comparisons and provides a diagnosis or procedure language for clinicians and other management staff.

Set against this, however, the disadvantages are considerable.

- Principally, the information is only as good as the base data input, which often lacks detail of severity, quality of care, dependency and outcome.

- All data provided by a hospital needs validation in the practice context. While hospitals can often analyse the most specific of conditions or surgical procedures, this level of information is too detailed for overall planning as there is insufficient aggregation.

The first of these points is one that cannot be overemphasized!

Information for managing the practice business

Information is valuable as an indicator of the health of the practice. The distinction between information and its sources must be borne in mind, ie the difference between what the practice staff want to know and where to go to find it. It is also important to recognize the importance of comparisons between different parts of the practice, between different periods of time and with other practices as a means of assessing performance.

Running a business has parallels with a patient consultation:

- presentation/review of a problem (history-taking)
- assimilation by the business of all the relevant facts (diagnosis)
- formulation of a management plan (prognosis/management plan)
- encouraging the recipient to accept the plan (patient compliance).

Patients may provide the doctor with a bewildering array of symptoms and complaints from which to choose. The doctor has been trained to sift the important from the less important; to put a hierarchy on the information; and to reassure, treat, or arrange immediate expert care. The doctor also uses information that currently exists in the patient's notes to try and make more sense of the symptoms and signs that are being presented.

The medical record equates with the history of the business – it is the baseline from which planning can take place.

Financial planning

Some of the symptoms and signs of a financially unhealthy practice are shown in Box 3.3. The financial performance of a practice, and hence its strength or vulnerability, is a critical indicator to the partners. One warning, however, is to have a healthy disrespect for the reliability of the data – Disraeli's comment about 'lies and damned lies' is perhaps appropriate here!

Sources of information include:

- the latest practice accounts (profit and loss statements, balance sheets)
- monthly management reports
- accounts.

The following should be considered:

- the availability and accuracy of the figures
- how long they take to produce
- whether they are on time

Box 3.3 Common symptoms and signs of an unhealthy practice

- Over-concentration on profit at the expense of cash flow
- Financing long-term investments with short-term money, eg financing a cost-rent scheme on an overdraft
- In constant arrears on tax/loans/hire purchase etc
- Increasing 'debtor collection' period, eg failure to meet FHSA claim deadlines, meaning that pay for work done is not received as soon as it could
- Continually failing to make a profit
- Management over-concerned with physical surroundings and trivia
- Regular desire to change bank/accountants

- who gets them
- how they are used.

There should be a short written commentary to monthly reports, and financial and cash flow forecasts explaining the ratios and comparisons with other practices.

An important point to consider is what questions should be asked. It is essential to identify trends by reference to historical data and an exception analysis of changing ratios. Practice liquidity should be assessed in terms of availability of funds and how highly geared (the relative proportion of loan to equity capital) the practice is. Such considerations provide an opportunity to review procedures and controls, risk and exposure, and alternative sources of income. These concepts are explained elsewhere[1]. The omission of examples of profit and loss statements, balance sheets and cash flow forecasts from this section is deliberate, because it is necessarily detailed and would detract from the development of the *principles* of obtaining information for practice management.

References

1.   Dean J (1994) *Making sense of practice finance, second edition.* Radcliffe Medical Press, Oxford.

4 | Business Planning and Human Resource Management

Business planning can materially enhance the capacity of a practice to manage its most valuable resource – its staff – more effectively. By providing a framework for linking individual activity to practice goals and a mechanism for monitoring that activity, inefficient duplication of activities can be reduced and much untapped staff potential released. The benefits to an organization of having effective staff management policies are shown in Box 4.1.

The quality of any organization depends crucially on the people working in it. The staff employed in a practice, and those attached to it, are the practice's most expensive resource. The challenge for doctors as employers is to turn this disparate collection of individuals into an enthusiastic and productive team, working together to achieve corporate goals.

The business plan is the starting point from which to begin meeting this challenge, because it articulates the agreed goals of the practice. The very process of producing the plan can, as discussed in Chapter 1, clarify the practice goals for the team and thus help them to appreciate the way in which their individual work activities can contribute to the achievement of these goals.

Although the business plan is a necessary prerequisite, it is insufficient in itself to prioritize the activities of the staff on a day-to-day basis. Box 4.2 outlines the sequence of key stages in the process of using the

---

Box 4.1 Advantages of an effective management policy

- Enjoyable place to work
- Attractive to potential employees
- Easier to manage because goals, objectives and standards have been set

---

Box 4.2   Business planning for effective human resource management

- Identifying key practice goals for the next 3–5 years
- Setting individual objectives
- Setting performance standards
- Identifying skills needed to perform activities to set standards
- Mapping staff competences (existing skills) against skills needed
- Developing training opportunities to help staff acquire missing skills
- Developing a performance appraisal process
- Developing an appropriate recognition strategy

---

business plan as a tool for developing effective staff management policies and procedures. These eight steps make up the process by means of which the practice can produce effective staff recruitment, training and development procedures, which serve to channel staff activities towards achieving the organization's potential.

Identifying key practice goals

The business plan provides the aims and goals to which the practice team has agreed to work. This has been discussed in detail in Chapter 1.

Setting objectives

The next management task is to provide the framework that supports the individual members of the team and allows them to carry out their own work in a way that contributes to the fulfilment of the goals. Setting clear objectives is the first stage of this process.

For example, one of the practice goals over the next 3–5 years might be to maximize its income from fees for item of service claims. One route towards this could lie in improving the take-up of cytology services among 45–55-year-olds. To achieve this practice objective, the partners might in turn set the practice nurses an objective: that of achieving a 30% increase in take-up by women in this age group within the following 12 months. In response to this objective, the practice nurses might decide to set up an additional clinic session specifically targeted at women of this age group. Although the nurses may be correct in their assumption that the provision of additional services will automatically lead to the desired result, that assumption needs further investigation before it becomes enshrined in practice policy.

This sort of investigation into a range of options can best be facilitated by tailoring the objective to suit the specific roles of each member of the team. This will help to ensure, for example, that the health visitor's skills are brought to bear on solving a problem in a way that does not duplicate the role of the practice nurse but complements it. Similarly, the practice manager and reception staff could be involved in monitoring the take-up of the additional clinic session and in notifying patients of the availability of the new service. Marketing the clinic should also include eliciting patients' reactions to it and any aspects of care that they would like to see incorporated into it.

Box 4.3 outlines how a practice objective can be translated into concrete and realistic objectives for individual members of the practice team. Such a process enables individual effort to be focused so that the corporate goal can be achieved. Each of the objectives detailed in Box 4.3 is aimed at focusing the activity of each individual towards the achievement of a specific aspect of the overall practice objective, yet each objective also reflects the individual areas of professional competence. Although the individual objectives should reflect expertise, they should not be too prescriptive and should be phrased in such a way that

---

Box 4.3   Setting objectives – a worked example

Practice goal: to maximize income from item of service fees

	Time-scale	Review periods
Practice objective To reach higher target for cytology	12 months	Quarterly

Practice manager's objective
   To establish mechanisms to
   improve cytology take-up
	12 months	Quarterly

Practice nurse's objective
   To increase take-up of cytology
   among the target population
	12 months	Quarterly

Receptionist's objective To operate administrative systems	1 month	Weekly
To identify and recall patients in the target group	3 months	Weekly

professional judgement and initiative can still be exercised in choosing the precise actions that will be taken to meet the objective set.

It can also be seen from the above example that the timescale for review of progress is not set arbitrarily, but varies according to the activity being performed. Certain activities must be in place and completed before others can start; these activities may need to be reviewed more frequently than others.

Finally, when practice and individual objectives are set, it must be remembered that only things that can be counted can be measured. To make sense to the practice and be understood by the staff, the objectives must be SMART, that is:

- specific

- measurable

- achievable

- realistic

- time-limited.

Setting performance standards

Once clear objectives have been set, the next step is to decide on the standard of performance required from each staff member in pursuit of the stated objective. To continue the earlier example, the practice nurse's objective is 'to increase the take-up of cytology among the target population' within 12 months, to be reviewed quarterly. Discussions with the practice nurse should be held to agree appropriate standards of activity to reach the stated objective. The activity in this case might be to set up a well woman clinic, and the required standards could be:

- to provide a service that attracts a 10% increase in patients attending for cytology tests in the first month and a further 10% increase in the second month

- to provide a service that meets professional guidelines of 'good practice'.

Setting specific objectives and then agreeing with the individual staff members standards to which the activity in pursuit of the objectives should be performed helps staff to focus their own efforts. Knowing the standards of performance expected of them enables staff to improve their efforts and also helps managers to give recognition to staff for reaching the set standard, both of which are key components of motivating staff.

Identifying skills needed to perform activity to set standards

Another advantage of structuring objectives and performance standards is that it helps managers to identify any gaps in skills that need to be filled if practice objectives are to be met. For example, the practice nurse may be confident working with a GP in cytology sessions, but does not feel happy about setting up her own clinic because she is aware that she lacks the appropriate training and experience. Agreeing objectives and standards provides a mechanism by which such skills gaps can be identified, which in turn can justify any additional training expenditure to be committed to fill the gaps.

Mapping staff competences against skills needed

Once the practice team has identified the skills that are necessary for the performance of specific activities, they are then in a position to determine the extent to which the team's existing skills meet the requirements. It may be, for example, that the practice nurse has received the necessary theoretical training in cytology testing techniques, but has not yet had practical experience, perhaps due to the lack of locally available, appropriate training.

Developing training opportunities

Identifying the gap in skills opens the door to finding alternative ways of filling it, eg by arrangement with a community clinic to provide supervised practical cytology work.

Setting standards of performance for activity at work helps managers to target training expenditure where it is most relevant for individual needs and for the practice objectives. Being clear about who needs what training and why enables managers to choose the most appropriate and cost-effective options. In some cases, developing in-house training may be the most appropriate solution; at other times an external course may be the only solution. In this event, however, the practice manager has the necessary information to ensure that the training course purchased reflects the practice's needs and priorities.

This process helps the practice to move away from a purely knowledge-based approach towards one that focuses on the acquisition of knowledge to support new skills. By concentrating expenditure on training that is matched to the practice goals identified in the business plan, the practice is prevented from falling into the trap of providing training for training's sake, or simply because a staff member has requested it and/or is available.

Performance appraisal

Having set both team and individual objectives, mechanisms are required to monitor and review at regular intervals the activity performed to meet the objectives. This enables any variations from the expected progress to be identified at an early stage, thus helping the practice to take early remedial action to avoid costly errors or omissions.

An effective performance appraisal scheme can:

- encourage staff to strive to improve their performance

- provide a cyclical mechanism by which objectives can be agreed, standards of performance set and performance measured, monitored and reviewed objectively

- allow recognition of achievement.

In all organizations, an appraisal system provides a framework for routine review of activity. Very often in small organizations, staff feel that they do not need a formal review process because they know each other very well. This 'knowledge' is often rather superficial, however, and such interactions as do exist may leave little opportunity for discussion of deeper, more personal staff concerns. The appraisal process facilitates open and honest disclosure of personal strengths and weaknesses in a constructive and supportive context. This kind of dialogue helps to create a good match between jobs to be filled and the range of skills available in the practice team.

Most people perform best when they are clear about what is expected of them and the standard against which their work will be judged. A performance appraisal scheme provides an *objective* framework for evaluating performance, and thus avoids judging work on the basis of the subjective criteria that are often used automatically. A good appraisal system will evaluate:

- individual performance
- how well the practice supports staff activity.

The annual cycle of objective setting and review incorporates opportunities for staff to identify any organizational constraints on individual performance. The extent to which the practice management can respond positively to such a challenge is a good indicator of the credibility of the scheme. How far the appraisal scheme is linked to pay and promotion rather than to staff development also affects its credibility and value to staff.

Setting up and implementing an effective appraisal scheme is a very demanding management activity. Further guidance on this complex but valuable aspect of staff management can be found elsewhere[1].

Recognition strategies

'Nothing succeeds like success' may be true, but only for a short while. Individuals at all levels in an organization crave recognition for work performed well. In Western societies, performance at work is a crucial component of an individual's sense of worth. Evidence of the converse can be seen daily in patients attending doctors' surgeries in areas where economic recession results in redundancies. Unfortunately, most employers have a tendency to criticize mistakes and lapses in performance more often than they praise successful activity.

Developing effective mechanisms for providing adequate recognition and reward has been a particularly thorny problem for the public sector generally and for the NHS in particular, with its reliance on central wage negotiations. Performance-related pay has been tried and found wanting within the NHS, though this has not yet led to its abandonment. Practices are at liberty, however, to set up their own performance-related pay schemes, which it is hoped can avoid the least successful aspects of the system. The following points should be considered in devising a recognition strategy.

- The main problem with financially related rewards as they currently exist within the NHS is the crudity of the system.

- Another problem of performance-related pay from an individual point of view is that money is a very short-lived incentive. Most people forget, or take for granted, their autumn pay rise by January, by which time they are looking for other evidence of recognition from their employer.

- Some practices are experimenting with practice manager partners.

- In the USA, health care organizations are also experimenting with staff share schemes, through which employees can benefit from the practice's increased productivity and prosperity, with encouraging results[2].

Whatever scheme is chosen, the evidence so far indicates that an effective staff reward scheme correlates strongly with the practice's overall success[2].

References

1. Irvine S and Haman H (1993) *Making sense of personnel management.* Radcliffe Medical Press, Oxford.

2. Private communication.

5 | Audit as a Component of Planning

Having looked at the theory behind business planning as applied to general practice, it is now time to turn to the practical application of these skills. At this point many GPs and practice managers will give up, bewildered by the vast array of problems that need to be solved, and uncertain of which to choose and where to start. Audit is a useful mechanism here.

One of the themes of this book is that progress in all areas will inevitably be slow; it is better to have gradual change with which all the staff will be able to cope, rather than sweeping away existing structures, losing the good as well as the bad and starting all over again. Evolution rather than revolution is the best way forward.

Each partnership must decide how much of its resources it will devote to the process of planning and change. Resources are of two basic types:

- financial
- effort/time.

It is one of the truisms of modern industrial society that those institutions and companies that fail to invest in new capital and plant will eventually become uncompetitive and fail. This is only partially true of general practice at the present time.

Financial resources

A substantial part of the income of a practice is derived not from activity but by existence. Capitation fees and deprivation payments merely require that the practice is open, not that it meets any particular stand-ards. Target fees together with health promotion income, however, do demand that the practice achieves the required standards in order for the remuneration to be gained. In purely financial terms, the difference between existence and activity will determine where the effort of the practice should first be placed.

The income from target schemes and health promotion can be calculated, and thus so can the return on any financial investment that is made to achieve them. The most obvious example in this context is employment by the practice of a nurse. If her sole tasks are related to enhancing the uptake of services so that targets and bandings can be achieved, the new income minus her salary (non-reimbursed portion) is, broadly speaking, the profit.

Effort and time

It is much more difficult to measure the impact of the amount of time and effort that should be devoted to the practice by the partners. There are no obvious parameters apart from the achievement of the minimal standards that are required. These consist of the following:

- Under the cost-rent scheme, practice development visiting teams inspect the premises to check that they meet the minimal requirements, eg for space, privacy and access for the disabled.

- Complaints by patients about the quality of service provided by the practice may eventually lead to a service committee. It is advantageous to have in place a practice scheme for the handling of suggestions and complaints by patients, and a sample is given in Appendix D.

- Independent medical advisers and eventually regional medical officers will offer advice and then impose sanctions if prescribing is 'way out of line' compared with the local norm.

What is audit?

Audit is the review of a process or behaviour to ensure that the proposed aims are being met.

- *Medical audit* is the review, undertaken by one or more practising doctors, of any aspect of medical care to ensure that proposed aims are being met.

- *Clinical audit* is the review, undertaken by one or more health professionals, to ensure that the proposed aims are being met.

- *Administrative audit* is the review, undertaken by health care professionals and/or staff of the administrative system, to ensure that the proposed aims are being met.

Who can undertake audit?

Those in a position to undertake audit are the members of the primary health care team. Once this simple statement has been made, it is necessary to define the team members within primary care (*see* Box 5.1)

Who should organize audit?

The power structure of a conventional organization consists of a chairman at the top, with managing director, divisional director and departmental managers below in ordered sequence. The implication is that the power resides at the top, and that instructions flow down while information flows up to where it is audited.

Box 5.1   Members of the primary health care team

Internal clinical	Doctors (GPs)
	Practice nurses
	District nurses
	Health visitors
	Midwives
	Others, eg psychologist, physiotherapist, chiropodist
Internal administrative	Receptionist
	Practice manager
	Business manager
	Secretary
Internal other	Patients
	Social workers
External contractual	FHSA
	Medical audit advisory groups
	Inland Revenue
External other	Consultants
	Other GPs
	Accountant

As discussed earlier, within primary care there are different types of audit: medical (involving only GPs); clinical (involving GPs and other health professionals); and administrative (involving health professionals and managers). The organization of audit in this context can be a complex process, and involves reference to the audit cycle:

- planning the data to be collected
- setting standards
- implementing action
- collecting data again
- resetting standards.

It is likely that even within one practice audit will simultaneously take place at different levels about different topics. It would be naïve to believe that only doctors can organize audit within a practice, and many nursing and administrative staff have carried out audit successfully.

Components of audit

It is possible to audit any business, including a general practice, in one of three different ways:

- structure
- process
- outcome.

Structure

Structure refers to the buildings, machines and people who work within an organization. If economists are to be believed, it is lack of investment within the structure of businesses that it is at the root of current economic problems. Investment in structure means building new premises or improving existing ones; it means buying new equipment; it also means employing new and additional staff.

All of these observations are applicable to general practice. There has been a recent boom in the building of new surgeries (possibly before the cash limiting of funds). Practices have been encouraged to computerize and to take on new staff, both to run the machines and to increase the range of services that are available.

Process

Process

Process refers to what happens within the premises. It is a description of the use to which the equipment is put; it also describes the activities of the employees.

Hundreds of processes take place within a general practice. They may be predominantly clinical or administrative. Each process can be broken down into a series of tasks that form the process. An example of this is when a patient telephones for an appointment.

- The telephone is answered.
- The call is diverted to the appointment book – optional.
- The type of appointment, when, and whether doctor/nurse is required is ascertained, and whether it is urgent/unbooked/routine.

Each of these tasks can be examined in detail and compared to any standards that have been decided.

- How many rings before the telephone is answered?
- Does the receptionist answer the telephone in a standard way?
- Where is the call dealt with? Is there a delay? Is the switchboard jammed?
- Are there enough appointments available in each of the given categories?
- Can urgent patients be seen that day?
- Can unbooked patients be seen in 24 hours?
- When is the next appointment with a named doctor or nurse?

This, of course, is the very stuff of audit. It is important to note that it is easier to audit process than either structure or outcome. This is, as noted above, because process can be split into manageable component parts.

Outcome

Outcome

Outcome in manufacturing industry is measured by the number of widgets that are made. If there are quality specifications for the widgets, these can be used to record a measure of productivity for the firm.

In a service industry such as medicine, it is much more difficult to measure outcome. In a few instances, eg immunization, process and outcome have become indistinguishable. In other words, it is assumed that immunization is universally a 'good' thing with a 100% positive outcome. This means that the process of immunization is what is counted. In order to qualify for target payments the GP has to prove that the patient has been immunized, not that the patient has seroconverted.

How do we know whether the outcome of our work either exists or is beneficial? This is a tricky area. One of the newer concepts that has been introduced to try and measure outcome is that of *health gain*. In essence, this is a concept devised by health planners who are attempting to measure the benefit for the population of any given intervention. Health gain is discussed further in Chapter 7.

Coarse audit

Coarseness as defined by Michael Green in his famous series *The Art of Coarse . . .* is not so much an attribute of people as of life towards people. It has nothing to do with spilling your gravy or eating your peas with a knife. Some tests of coarseness in everyday life are given in Box 5.2.

Mr Green gives many examples in his book. He defines a coarse actor as one who knows his lines but not necessarily the order in which they come, and the coarse sailor as one who in a crisis shouts, 'For God's sake turn left!' On this basis, the authors' definition of a coarse GP is 'one who decides what to treat the patient with and then makes a diagnosis fit'.

By an extension of this concept, coarse audit is a method of evaluating activity within a practice, attempting to refer it to the accepted normal standard. The synonyms of 'evaluate' can be considered threatening and include the words: grade, score, rate, judge, verify, assess, estimate and rank. All of these words suggest that the performance of the practice in a certain area will be scrutinized and compared with what is going on elsewhere among the practice's peers. The synonyms of 'normal', however, are far more comforting. They include the following words: customary, habitual, standard, established, common, unimpressive, typical, everyday, mundane, unexceptional and unremarkable. This list is far more comforting because it emphasizes that most practices will be normal, they will be typical, and that practices do not have to strain and strive for excellence in all activities that they undertake; they merely have

---

Box 5.2   Everyday examples of coarseness

- Do shop assistants go on talking when you want to pay?

- When you cash a cheque at a bank, do they go to see if there is any money in your account?

- Do bar staff look at you and then serve the person standing directly behind you?

to make sure that their standards have reached a mark that is acceptable amongst their peers.

Standards

There are perhaps four standards against which practices can rate themselves, as follows.

- Gold: a gold standard is when success, however that is measured, reaches the maximum obtainable in today's climate. By its very nature, a gold standard can only be reached by a few pioneers in a certain area, and it is unlikely that any one practice would be able to reach gold standards in more than one area. It often happens that the emphasis that is placed on, and the resources that are put into, the effort to reach a gold standard may detract from work in other areas.

- Normal: this is what typically goes on in practices. It is initially defined by measuring what happens today in a cross-section of practices. It may subsequently be decided that normal practice should be improved by setting standards and that a typical practice should be able to then attain the new standard. This, however, is inevitable, because as practices achieve the standards set for them, the normal standards will continually improve.

- Minimal: it is ever more likely that minimal criteria will be applied to aspects of primary health care. This is already happening in an administrative sense, eg practice development visiting teams assessing the suitability of practice premises. Minimal standards imply that in order for the practice to be accepted, it must remain above this standard, though it may fall below normal.

- Unacceptable: this is a continuation of the above process, whereby if the practice falls below the minimal standard this is not accepted. In the example of the practice development visiting team, rent and rate reimbursement may be withheld.

If a practice decides that it is a coarse general practice, then coarse audit holds no fears for it. There is no need to try and attain a gold standard, merely to keep the practice above minimal standards in all the areas that are being audited, particularly those areas that are examined by external bodies, eg the FHSA.

If, however, the practice is made aware by the increasing activity of audit of the normal standards throughout its peer practices (and this undoubtedly will be a function of the medical audit advisory groups), the goal should be to stay within or to attain that standard. The practice should also not be disappointed to find, when it has reached the standard, that new standards have been set.

Practice audit: a practical example

Coarse audit

The following example of a coarse audit relates to a fundholding aspect of the authors' practice, but could equally apply to a non-fundholding practice. This is a summary of events that took place over an 18-month period, in which a new physiotherapy service for patients was established in conjunction with the Priority Services Group at Whitchurch Hospital, Cardiff.

The aim was to improve physiotherapy services to the patients. The objectives were:

* to determine current services
* to agree appropriate outcome measures
* to agree a new system
* to re-audit.

An audit of physiotherapy referrals was carried out as a baseline. The data obtained (Box 5.3) were sparse and had many flaws and gaps, typical of a retrospective audit. The collection of data of this type poses as many questions as it provide answers, and to some extent this is its main value.

Useful information in assessing provision of services

It is essential in the process of audit to identify the questions to be answered and how. Some questions relevant to the above coarse audit are given below.

* Is the waiting time for patients to be seen for a first appointment known?

There was no accurate information within the practice, though it was felt to be 4–6 weeks at that time. This can be easily recorded.

* Can the non-attendance rate be reduced from the present level of 32% at the first appointment?

This can be routinely recorded.

Box 5.3   Coarse retrospective audit of physiotherapy referrals, 1990

100 sets of notes out of 121 referrals were audited; nine patients were referred for aids and have been excluded from the rest of the audit.

91 patients; 57 female, 34 male

Mean age, 46 years (range, 19–84 years)

Mean number of consultations before referral, 3.5 (range, 1–10)

Diagnoses
Back pain/sciatica	46
Neck pain	16
Shoulder pain	14
Osteoarthritic knee	3
Miscellaneous	12

Referring doctor
A	18
B	15
C	14
D	11
E	10
F	6
G	4
H	2
?	1

Radiography
Sciatica	21
Shoulder	4
Neck	3
Osteoarthritis	2
Other	2

Outcome after receiving physiotherapy
Better	28 (31%)
No better	9 (10%)
Unclear	25 (27%)
Did not attend for appointment	29 (32%)

Treatments given
	Traction
	Exercises (including McKenzie)
	Back-school
	Ultrasound
	Pulsed short-wave diathermy
	Heat

- Is it known what happens to patients when they are seen? How many are given advice? How many need active treatment?

This is amenable to a prospective study within the physiotherapy department.

- Do the patients get better?

This can be measured both subjectively and objectively and by both the patients and the caring professionals. Patients can be asked to rate the effectiveness of their treatment, and measures such as the ability to return to work or resume domestic chores can be assessed. The physiotherapy department can also give a view of the severity of disability of the patient at the beginning and end of treatment.

- Do the patients approve of the service?

This is amenable to a prospective satisfaction survey.

Pilot scheme

Following the coarse audit, a pilot scheme to improve the physiotherapy service provided was started on 1 April 1991. The main points in its design were the following.

- Patients were made aware that the initial assessment by a physiotherapist would take place in the surgery.

- A physiotherapist from Whitchurch Hospital attended for a morning session (9.30–12.30 am) initially every 2 weeks. Appointments were available for six patients to be seen at each session (approximately 150/year). If demand altered then the sessions could be adjusted accordingly.

- The appointment book was held at the surgery. Written referrals were placed with the practice receptionist for the attention of the physiotherapist.

- The cost of maintaining the support service at the surgery was borne by the doctors.

- If the patient was deemed to require further treatment, this was carried out at Whitchurch Hospital. An attempt was made to inform the patient of the likely time of the appointment during the assessment session. The physiotherapist completed the referral letter for each patient seen. Each patient completed a satisfaction survey.

- If radiographs were deemed necessary by the physiotherapist, they were authorized by the GP.

- After the course of treatment was completed, the physiotherapist sent out a standard letter. At this point, the patient was also asked to complete the final satisfaction survey.

- It was necessary for both the doctors and the rest of the primary health care team to meet with the physiotherapist on a regular basis during this pilot stage, so that the initial results could be fed back and flaws and problems with the system ironed out.

- The intention was that the service should be manned continuously, so that sickness or annual leave was covered whenever possible.

Audit of physiotherapy referrals

The audit of the scheme from April to October 1991 is shown in Box 5.4, and the summary of the audit in Box 5.5.

Box 5.4 Audit of physiotherapy referrals in the pilot scheme, April–October 1991

Number of referrals to screening clinic, 127

Number of community visits, 2

Outcome measures

Full recovery	17
Optimal potential reached	21
Improved – further improvement expected	31
Improved – no further improvement expected	6
Only required advice at screening clinic	11
Worse due to other factors	4
No change	12
Transferred elsewhere	3
Only attended screening clinic, no outcome	8
Did not attend (Whitchurch)	6
Did not attend (screening clinic)	2
Did not complete treatment, no outcome	6

Screening clinic
19 (15%) of patients attended this part of the service only

Advice given	11
Inappropriate referrals	5
Already recovered	2
Would not travel to Whitchurch	1

Patients' views

A postal survey of 81 patients who attended Whitchurch was carried out, and a response rate of 33% was achieved.

- 67% of patients found the service helpful.
- 55% of patients thought they were better.
- 7% thought they were worse.
- 52% of patients had no problem in getting to Whitchurch.
- 33% found it difficult; two buses are required from Ely to Whitchurch.

Has useful information been gained?

At this point the original questions posed at the start of the project should be considered.

- Is the waiting time for patients to be seen for a first appointment known?

Before: there was no accurate information in the practice, though it was felt to be 4–6 weeks at that time.
After: the median waiting time for the appointment was 11 days.

- Can the non-attendance rate be reduced from the present level of 32% at the first appointment?

Yes – the non-attendance rate for the first appointment during the audit was 3%. It is now running at 8%.

- Is it known what happens to patients when they are seen?

Those given advice, 15%.
Those needing active treatment, 85%.

- Do the patients get better?

83% showed some improvement.

- Do the patients approve of the service?

Box 5.5 Summary of outcomes in the pilot physiotherapy scheme

	A	B	C	D	E	F	Total	Mean number of attendances
Back	0	8	2	9	10	9	38	5.7
Neck	1	1	0	7	2	1	12	4.1
Shoulder	0	1	1	5	7	4	18	6.5
Knee/ankle	2	1	0	5	1	2	11	4.9
Other	0	1	3	4	0	1	9	6.4
Total	4	12	6	31	21	17	91	

Key: A, worse due to factors other than treatment (4%); B, no change (13%); C, improved, but not as before illness or injury – no further improvement expected (7%); D, improved, but not as before illness or injury – further improvement expected (34%); E, optimal potential reached (23%); F, full recovery made (18%).

The patients' questionnaire was limited. The anecdotal feedback from patients still ranges from very positive to neutral, but negative comments are few. No further changes have been made to the system.

An administrative audit has just been completed in order to identify how information may be better recorded and retrieved.

6 | Planning for a Patient-centred Practice

In order to plan for a patient-centred practice, the practice needs information about its patients, their characteristics and needs. This is the practice *market*, which includes both potential and existing patients. Gathering information about them is *market research*, and by knowing the type and range of services they need and want it is possible for the practice to 'market' the services it provides to mutual benefit. The types of questions that can then be answered include the following.

- What is the optimum list size for the practice?

- Is the list size increasing, decreasing or static?

- Does the practice qualify for deprivation payments?

- Is the level of contraceptive fees what is expected?

Marketing is the process of planning and executing the conception, pricing, promotion and distribution of ideas, goods and services to create exchanges that satisfy individual and organizational objectives. No service that the practice provides will be taken up by patients unless there is a demand for it. The demand is constituted by the group of individuals, patients or potential patients, who make up the market for that particular service. For example, patients with a need for diabetic care are only a small proportion of the total list size, constituting a *segment* of the population. A diabetic clinic in the practice is a waste of resources unless the need for it either exists or can be created. Breaking down the practice population into discrete groups is technically referred to as *market segmentation*.

Market segmentation is the division of a total market into two or more parts, where each part exhibits relatively similar needs and wants for a particular product/service and thus require different marketing strategies. The market can be considered as the practice patients or the residents of the practice locality. These markets can then be broken down into specific groups or segments, based on:

- the identifiable characteristics of towns, cities, localities and counties
- the patterns by which patients live and care for their health
- the identifiable characteristics of individual patients.

The marketing concept starts with an assessment of patient needs and wants, deciding which needs to meet, and thus achieving practice goals through patient satisfaction. The benefits of segmentation include:

- improved allocation of health care resources
- better identification of service opportunities
- guidelines for development of district strategies for target segments
- improved product/service positioning relative to consumer needs and competition
- provision of further guidelines for product/service developments.

The steps in planning a practice segmentation strategy are shown in Box 6.1.

Marketing health services

This section is intended to contribute to the practice's understanding of marketing within the strategic planning process, by applying general

---

Box 6.1   Steps in planning a practice segmentation strategy

- Determining the characteristics and needs of patients for the product or service
- Analysing patient similarities and differences
- Developing patient group profiles
- Selecting patient segment(s)
- Positioning the practice's offering in relation to competition
- Establishing an appropriate marketing plan

marketing concepts to the health care system. To this extent, marketing is the process that provides the fit or link between three aspects:

- the potential needs and wants of the marketplace
- the environmental opportunities and constraints
- the intrinsic skills and available resources of the organization.

Just as a coin has two sides, there are two complementary approaches to marketing.

- An inside-out approach will determine what specific attributes possessed by the practice could be attractive to others to use.
- An outside-in analysis will examine the environment within which the practice operates, to identify any latent demand ready to be expressed by the patient for services that are yet to be established.

Marketing strategy and process

The starting point for an effective marketing strategy, within an overall strategic planning process, is to identify the exact nature of patients' wants and needs. It will then be possible to take meaningful decisions as to which needs the practice is willing and able to meet and which will allow the practice to achieve its organizational goals through enhanced patient satisfaction. When identifying the wants and needs of the patients, the practice must be conscious of the personal, cultural, psychological and social factors that influence patient behaviour. It must be borne in mind that general practices are now operating in a competitive market-place, and the comparative patient response to the strategies adopted by the practice and its competitors could be critical to success.

Too often in health care, there is no attempt to target specific patient groups. This is possibly a response of services that are in general sought by the population as a whole, to a greater or lesser extent. It should be remembered that the quality of data about patient needs (as opposed to wants) is not always good, and this makes the analysis of the market much harder. A practice may be able, however, to identify differences in its service provision compared with its competitors and that there is a need to implement a segmentation strategy.

Planning the segmentation strategy

The practice must determine the characteristics of the patient needs in different market segments for its health care services and products, and analyse the similarities and differences thus identified. Most general practices will be similar to provider hospitals in that they possess little sophistication in marketing within the practice, and an external resource may be necessary. The steps in planning the segmentation strategy are:

- development of patient group profiles that will allow patient segments to be selected; it is important that all those involved in the marketing exercise agree on the variables by which the segments will be identified, otherwise the patient group profiles will have no common validity

- evaluation of the attractiveness of each segment in relation to the overall strategic plan of the practice

- selection of the segments to be targeted

- determination and development of the position for each target segment.

In the positioning process, the relevant set of comparative products (in this case, products and services provided by the practice and its competitors) are examined. In order to depict the positioning of products in graphical format, it is necessary to predefine the criteria that constitute the axes of the graph. Each of the products being considered will have particular attributes or characteristics that help to distinguish it from the others. Those attributes which are significant to the chosen criteria (the axes of the graph) – the determinant attributes – can be used to plot the position of each product. As an example, for the practice appointment system the timeliness (availability) of an appointment can be plotted against its specificity (chosen doctor). Both patient preferences and current service provision can be plotted on the same axes (Figure 6.1), for one or more practices. From this, a 'need' can be identified and a potentially attractive service devised for the benefit of both the practice and the patients.

It also follows that 'competitor' practice profiles must be examined to establish:

- what levels and quality of services they offer

- how they attract new patients

- their attitudes to competition

- the partner profiles (dynamic/expansionist or ageing/reactive/traditionalist)

- their relative success.

It will then be possible to collect information from both patients and potential patients about each product based on these determinant at-

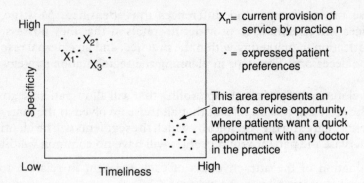

Figure 6.1   Positioning of a product (service) in the market.

tributes. The intensity of the product's current position in the patient's mind can be analysed. This allows the product 'space' to be clearly defined in relation to the patient's expressed and most preferred combination of the determinant attributes, which gives a good measure of the market position.

Detailed analysis can then be performed on the accuracy of fit between the market (preferences) position and the product position. It will then be possible for the practice to select and develop a positioning or repositioning strategy.

The marketing mix

Having identified the constituent segments of the market and taken account of the individual products and services of the practice, it is possible to establish the appropriate marketing 'mix' for each target segment in terms of the product, its price, method of promotion and distribution. An example is shown in Box 6.2. In determining the marketing mix, the team must be clear on their approach to:

- differentiation – distinguishing the product or potential product from those of competitors

- cost leadership – the price to consumers; in this context it is non-monetary, eg the price to the patient of a last-minute appointment is a consultation with a GP other than the usual one

- focusing on the product – the match between the product and patient's need/desires.

In health care, as elsewhere, each product has a life cycle in relation to technological and competitive change (Figure 6.2). The 'marketing team'

Box 6.2   Marketing mix for the development of a new product

- Product: the development of a 7.00 am surgery on weekdays
- Benefits:
  —patients do not need time off work
  —for the practice, having this as an unbooked surgery will reduce demand at the peak time of 9.00–11.00 am
- Price:
  —patient has to get up earlier and queue
  —practice has staff and overhead costs to meet
- Promotion: time-effective to patients and reduces overall daily stress to partners and patients
- Place (distribution): the branch surgery, thus keeping costs low

---

in the practice should ensure that the product portfolio is such that several products are available at each stage of the cycle to allow total income to meet practice requirements.

Marketing decisions

This is a crucial area for the medical staff and management at the practice. The marketing plan will need to clearly specify:

- the speed and timing of the programme
- the number and identity of locations in which marketing takes place
- how far ahead of its competitors the practice is
- what measures will be used to assess success (gross revenue, service uptake etc)
- how the results will be applied to decide whether to extend a pilot scheme, modify the product, or withdraw it from the market.

In health care, the opportunities to affect pricing are relatively few, and other approaches are often needed to supplement the price strategy. This is because most services provided are NHS activity, which is free to the patient, and the income derived from the NHS is centrally fixed. The same is not true for income-earning private work. In establishing this, the practice will have to take account of:

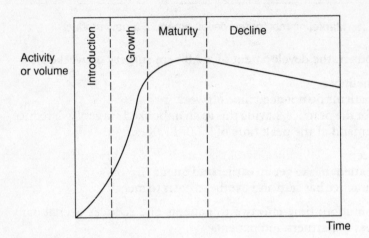

Figure 6.2   Life cycle of a product (service).

- its own cost considerations (margins, profit, break-even points)
- market demand considerations (loyalty of patients)
- competition-based factors (price leadership, reaction to change, legality).

It should be recognized that marketing communications strategies are often difficult to implement in the health care area, as the budget available may not be sufficient to permit the widespread promotion that is necessary. Practices do not have the opportunity to advertise in the press (general or medical), television, radio, direct mailshots, or hoardings. Clearly, decisions must be made on:

- the budget available
- the exact message to be put across
- the most appropriate mechanism for marketing
- the nature of evaluation.

Full evaluation is not always possible, as the results in the health marketing context are complex to interpret.

Specific options for the practice

Some possible areas and issues for consideration by the marketing team are shown in Box 6.3. These are not exhaustive and are certainly not prescriptive. They and other issues have to be examined in the overall context of secondary services, where trends indicate:

- a reduction in total patient admissions
- shorter stays
- under-utilized departments
- seasonal variations in demand for service
- increasing complexity of technology (and consequent high capital charges).

Within primary care the practice should consider:

- the increased threats of competition from local practices and other professions
- more regulatory constraints
- FHSA inspections
- the balance between a commercial and a caring image
- the ability of management to reorient towards a marketing/cost–benefit/efficiency bias
- the manner in which the practice responds to threats and opportunities.

Box 6.3   Issues for consideration by the practice marketing team

- Possibilities for adoption/development of in-surgery diagnostic tests and procedures
- The impact of shifts from secondary to primary care on overall service provision
- The characteristics of the practice population and of the local area
- The experience of clinicians and their involvement in continuing medical education
- Changes in practice-based services over the last 3 years and any developments by the competition
- Concerns of consultants towards the development in out-patient care with reference to primary health care provision

---

The whole emphasis should be to focus on value-added services to the patient.

Should the practice market itself?

There are a number of obstacles to effective marketing of health care. It is often conceived to be unethical, irrelevant and catering to artificially created demand. Sometimes it is thought to be too exotic or expensive and nothing more than selling and advertising. This may be a result of initial efforts in the field of health care marketing, which emphasized the caring aspects and detailed doctors and facilities, but failed to offer solutions to patient problems.

Effective health care marketing can achieve the following.

• It leads to a better understanding of individual patient segments of the practice and the market, which can differ markedly from one another.

• It allows existing services to be carefully shaped to need and new services to be responsive to a changing environment.

• By concentrating resources in the areas where the practice provides a strong and stable service through the use of more effective methods of delivery, a higher level of patient satisfaction can be achieved consistent with practice goals.

Some general practices are now beginning to apply marketing to a broader set of problems, in an attempt to answer critical questions such as:

• where should the practice locate a branch surgery?

• how can the practice estimate whether a new service will draw enough patients?

• what should a practice do with an asthma clinic that has only 20% uptake?

• how can the practice attract more patients to preventive care services, eg childhood immunization and cancer screening programmes?

• what marketing programmes can build practice goodwill and attract more patients?

Handling the media

When fundholding began, the first practices were very much in the limelight of the press. Becoming a fundholder no longer attracts such attention, but it is still important to be able to deal with the local media. They will certainly visit the practice if any changes to referral patterns are considered, particularly if a consultant takes umbrage!

There are two basic points to remember:

- always be prepared
- always tell the good news.

Any media interview can be used positively to promote the image of the practice. Inevitably, the media (newspapers, television, or radio) are looking for the controversial and the interesting. Any spokesperson must remember to give the practice viewpoint, not a personal opinion. The interview may be held on practice premises, by telephone (for newspaper and radio), or in a studio (for radio and television).

Adequate preparation requires the interviewee to know:

- the location of the interview
- the length of the interview
- who else is being interviewed
- whether it is a straight interview or a panel discussion
- whether there will be a live audience
- what approach the interviewer will take.

Nothing is better preparation than having a full command of the facts, and the practice team member is present as the 'expert'. The pregnant pause should be avoided at all costs. Throughout, it is important to focus entirely on the interviewer and not to get distracted by technicians or others moving in the background.

The interviewee should wear something comfortable and, if the interview is on television, think about the appropriate appearance to achieve (Box 6.4).

If the interviewer wants to talk about a topic for which the interviewee is not prepared, it is quite acceptable to say that this is not part of the brief and will not be discussed. Interviewers need to make interviews informative and entertaining for the viewer/reader, and often throw out challenging remarks to liven them up. It is therefore important to understand their techniques (and how to deal with them).

Box 6.4 Appropriate appearance for appearing on television interviews

- Choose clothes that reflect your professional image

- Do not wear clothes that are shiny, stiff, or boldly patterned, eg checks or stripes

- Avoid black, white and navy blue, as they do not photograph well

- Be careful of large amounts of red and yellow near the face, as these colours have a tendency to 'run' into the skin. Instead, wear pastel shades, eg beige, brown, grey, or green. Light colours also make you look younger

- Do not wear glittering jewellery. If if catches the television lights it can be very distracting; it is also noisy (this also applies to radio)

- Men should wear long socks (in case of a long shot)

- Women should wear skirts that are comfortable and do not ride up

- Let the make-up artist powder your face or bald spot to avoid shine

- Make sure you pull your jacket down and straighten your tie to give a neat, caring appearance

- Sit upright and be alert. Beware of the swivel chair. Do not swivel!

- Look positive, sit slightly forward, but try to appear natural

---

- They question credentials (so the facts must be known).
- They want to show off their own knowledge (so they should be praised).
- They cite new evidence (their sources should be asked for).
- They disagree with the interviewee (so again the facts must be known).

If the questioner interrupts, if possible the interviewee should pause until the end of the interruption and then continue with the answer, without trying to talk louder. If a question contains false information, it should be corrected before dealing with it. The audience will remain on the side of the interviewee provided that he/she:

- remains in control
- uses neutral and objective statements

- answers concisely
- never rises to the bait of a loaded question.

A summary of how to approach answering questions in any type of interview is given in Box 6.5.

Box 6.5 How to handle interviews

- Be assertive
- Nothing is 'off the record'
- Do not expect reporters to believe you
- Never lie
- Avoid saying 'no comment'
- Do not let reporters put words into your mouth
- Keep answers short and simple
- Do not use complex medical terms, jargon, lists, or too many numbers
- Do not give one word answers – use questions as prompts
- Be prepared for anything
- Get your view across, no matter what questions are asked
- Concentrate on the interviewer; ignore everything else
- Do not smoke or drink alcohol
- If you prefer not to discuss something, say so beforehand
- Never lose your temper; keep language neutral
- Do not be afraid of silence
- Prepare practice policy statements
- Be aware of body language
- Think positively and enjoy yourself

---

7 | Planning for Service Developments

The numerous processes that take place within the practice on a daily basis have already been alluded to in previous chapters. This chapter will look in detail at some examples. Within each process, the decisions taken on each individual component of that process will add up to the service that the patient (in business terms, the customer) will experience.

Appointments – systems and patients

One of the most commonly heard phrases in any general practice is: 'the appointment system is not working'. It is salutary to reflect on some of the phrases that are used by receptionists and their impact on the patients who are seeking to arrange health care from their GP. They include:

- 'there are no appointments left'
- 'we are fully booked'.

The area of arranging how patients see their GPs is one that is amenable to the principles of planning. Even before a baseline measurement of the current system, however, it is important to have a clear idea of the underlying objectives of any appointment system. The questions that need to be answered are shown in Box 7.1.

Consider the situation when no appointment system exists at all. In this situation the only constraint on the number of patients who may attend is time. In other words, the doors to the surgery are open for a fixed period. The patients know that if they attend during that 'window of opportunity' they will see the GP, though there is no indication of how long it will take before that time is reached.

The advantages of this system from the patient's point of view is that no advance planning is needed. This is particularly useful in cases of

---

Box 7.1 Basic considerations for an appointment system

- Who is the appointment system for, patients or doctors?
- What type of system is required? Booked, partially booked, extras, unbooked?
- What length of appointment is required?
- Are there different types of appointment?
- What plans are there for planned or unplanned absence?
- How will the system be judged?
- How will the number of appointments needed be calculated?

---

minor acute illness, because a patient can see a GP fairly soon after the onset of symptoms. The advantage of this system to the GP may lie elsewhere within the overall activity of the practice. The fact that patients can be seen without any formal barriers may mean a concomitant reduction in the number of house calls requested for patients with minor illness.

The disadvantage for the patient, of course, is the uncertainty of how many other patients will have turned up to see that GP on that day and therefore the waiting time to see the GP. The behaviour of the GP may also vary – from feeling under very slight pressure when the surgery is not busy to feeling under extreme pressure when there are 20 other patients still waiting to be seen.

If this system is postulated as having major disadvantages for the GPs in the sense that they have little control over their work-load, the implications of a rigid appointment system where each patient has to book in advance a slot to see the GP must be considered.

Advantages of booked appointments

From the patients' point of view, they have a clear idea of approximately when they are going to be seen, though it must be said that many appointment systems do not run to time. In fact, there appears to be an expectation among patients that there will be a degree of slippage. Nevertheless, in the age of the patients' charter, it is expected that patients will be seen within a certain time of their stated appointment or, if not, that an adequate and reasonable explanation will be given. The patients' charter for the authors' surgery is given in Appendix E.

This appointment system, of course, requires a degree of advance planning and also requires that patients understand at which stage during any given illness they need to take the initiative to book an appointment.

Disadvantages of booked appointments

The lack of flexibility from the patients' point of view means that it may be difficult to obtain an appointment, particularly with the GP of choice, within a time-scale that the patient considers acceptable. It is interesting to ponder on the full implications of the phrase 'there are no appointments left'.

The advantage to the GP of this system is that complete control is exercised over the number of patients that are seen in a set period of time, even if total control over the amount of work per patient is not necessarily predictable in advance. Nevertheless, with judgement and experience it should be possible for GPs to predict the number of patients they should see per hour in order to meet the demands that patients normally make on them.

It is inevitable in any system that there will be occasions when patient demands are such that the whole system breaks down, eg because one patient may require 30 min of the GP's time. One of the safeguards that has to be built in to any appointment system is to know how often this occurs and how it is dealt with.

Types of patient demand

In order to ensure a happy medium between the advantages of a fully unbooked system and the advantages of a rigidly booked system, the different types of patient must be recognized (Box 7.2).

The number of type 3 patients seen will depend on the number of appointments that are bookable, and also on whether the GP encourages patients to re-attend on a regular basis or leaves the choice to the patient's discretion. Other factors that impinge on this equation are the availability and utilization of practice nurses for the follow up and management of chronic conditions and the monitoring of patients by means of a repeat prescription register.

It is important at this stage to determine the objectives of each individual practitioner, and in a group practice also how a consensus can be reached, in order that quality standards for waiting times can be generated. Such criteria could be:

• how long patients have to wait to see any GP in the practice from the time of telephoning

---

Box 7.2   Different types of patient

- Type 1: those who want to see a GP – any GP – because they perceive that they have an urgent problem that requires rapid medical attention. These patients tend to be seen as 'extras' or in unbooked/emergency surgeries

- Type 2: those who wish to see any GP, but at a specific time and place – those who value an appointment

- Type 3: those who require follow up of a chronic or acute condition. These patients often value continuity of care and wish to see 'their' GP, whether the consultation is patient-initiated or GP-initiated

---

- how long patients have to wait from the time of telephoning if the problem is urgent

- how long patients have to wait to see the GP of their choice.

The GPs also have to look honestly at the effort and depth they give to a planned appointment compared with one that is perceived to be 'extra' to the basic appointment system.

- Are 'extras' viewed as patients in whom only the presenting complaint should be dealt with, or is the same amount of time and effort as with a planned appointment put into providing health promotion, chronic disease management etc?

- Should patients who attend for urgent appointments have problems that the GP deems to be urgent or that the patient deems to be urgent, eg is it reasonable for a patient who finds out that a sick note has expired to make an urgent appointment to see the GP?

Designing the appointment system

When all these issues have been clarified between the partners and a clear policy has been formulated, it is possible to look at the current system in order to see what inefficiencies exist. It may be possible to set up a hierarchy of aims as shown in Box 7.3.

At this point the GP or practice manager has to indulge in some mathematical calculations to understand the implications of setting these standards. It is necessary to have some idea of how many patients fall into

---

Box 7.3   Hierarchy of aims in setting up an appointment system

- All patients who request an urgent appointment with a non-named GP should be seen the same day

- All patients who request an appointment with a non-named GP should be seen within 24 hours

- All patients who request a planned appointment with a named GP should be seen within a defined, acceptable time

---

each of the categories defined above, against which can be set the total number of appointments available with all the GPs who work in the practice on a daily basis.

In the authors' practice the GPs consult at a rate of three patients/20 minutes for a surgery lasting 2 hours, giving a total of 18 patients seen in each surgery by each GP. The strategy to accommodate type 1 patients is as follows.

- The GP on call for the afternoon will see all patients who request an appointment up to the end of surgery – 6.00 pm. The number of patients seen in a consulting session varies, but is usually greater than the patients who would have been seen if that GP had been allocated 18 planned appointments.

- All other GPs have 50% of their 18 afternoon appointments allocated for type 1 patients. This means that with an average of five GPs consulting each afternoon, 60% of appointments are reserved for patients who wish to be seen that day.

- The GP who has been on call the night before will see all those patients who request to be seen that morning.

This last surgery also caters for type 2 patients who request an appointment with an unnamed GP within 24 hours. The demand for this 'combined' service certainly outstrips the 18 planned slots. This is accommodated by:

- asking patients to attend surgery from 9.15 am. Type 2 patients are given an appointment time, while type 1 are told that they will be seen as soon as possible

- letting the GP continue the surgery for as long as required.

In the last eventuality, this GP may not then be available to participate in house calls. If the work-load appears to be becoming too great for the individual GP, it is possible to divert other GPs from house calls to meet the demand within surgery.

The implications of meeting the stated quality standards in the authors' practice has been that as a general rule:

- all patients who request an urgent appointment with a non-named GP are seen the same day

- all patients who request an appointment with a non-named GP are seen within 24 hours

- all patients who request a planned appointment with a named GP will be seen as soon as possible.

If the number of planned appointments is insufficient, the consequence is that patients will complain that it is not possible to make a routine appointment with the GP of their choice within a time they consider reasonable. If this is so, the practice has two choices if it wishes to acquiesce:

- the number of appointments available can be increased

- the number of urgent 24-hour appointments can be reduced, so that the number of routine appointments is concomitantly increased.

There is no 'correct' solution to help with the balancing act between these two competing needs. The example that is given above is merely one solution. What is essential is that the practice members have a clear view of the desired outcome – of the service they are attempting to provide and to what standards. There are a number of factors to consider.

- There are always competing demands on GPs' time, and certainly GPs have been known to complain that patients abuse the system by saying they wish to be seen within 24 hours in order to obtain what the GPs perceive as care for minor problems.

- A policy of having non-named GPs for the urgent/24 hour service means that those patients who do value continuity of care, particularly for chronic conditions, can have their different aims and objectives met by a booked surgery rather than attending 'their GP' during an unbooked surgery.

- The number of routine appointments required is influenced by the frequency with which GPs ask patients with given conditions to return for review, and whether this review is carried out by the same GP or by another member of the practice team.

In particular, the practice nurse can monitor hypertension, diabetes, or asthma. If patients with hypertension are reviewed weekly, as opposed to 3-monthly, this obviously has a dramatic impact on the utilization of routine appointments, whether with the GP or the practice nurse. The way that patients are reviewed can vary greatly between individual GPs, and it is important that there is consensus and that guidelines are written in order to standardize care across the practice and to ensure that the practice partners feel that the system is being used fairly by the staff as well as by the patients.

Monitoring

The system can be monitored in the first instance by the receptionists, who have a very clear idea of, for example:

- when the next appointment is with a GP
- when the next urgent appointment is
- whether patients are being turned away because one of the GPs has a 3-week delay before any of his 'chronic patients' can book to see him.

If this information is collected in a standardized form and passed to either the practice manager or the practice partners, the system can be reviewed and changes can be implemented as necessary.

Absence of a practice team member

The absence of a practice team member means that a fixed number of appointments is removed from the system for a period of time. This may be on a planned basis (holidays) or an unplanned basis (sickness). When judging the impact of the removal of such appointments from the system, the principles on which the system runs have to be looked at again.

- Do the underlying quality criteria still stand?
- Will the same priority be given to the urgent or 24-hour appointments or will they be curtailed in order that the level of routine appointments can be maintained?
- Will the remaining partners work harder and longer to maintain the number of appointments during the absence?

The obverse of this coin is that when all partners are present, they may not have to work as hard as normal if the system is designed to run with allowance for planned absences.

Out-of-hours contacts

The number of telephone calls that it takes the patient to contact the GP is a quality issue. It is a part of the service that can be easily subjected to an external audit on a 24-hour basis.

FHSAs may stipulate that in order to conform to local patient charter standards, no more than two telephone calls should be made. If it is assumed that the first call will be to the surgery, the quality standard has been met if this is automatically forwarded to the answering service, GP's home, mobile, or deputizing service. If a recorded message is received on making the first call, the number given must then put the patient in touch with one of the above services.

Advantages of an answering service

The decisions made will affect the GP's family as well as the patient. Although many patients wish to speak to the GP, they are also happy to receive telephone advice on the best way to manage the current medical condition. Mobile phones and answering services have the advantage that they render the GP's family independent of the GP. In this age of technology, it appears anachronistic that spouses and children should be confined to home to provide a telephone answering service for the GP who is on call.

Disadvantages of an answering service

Answering services do have one drawback as far as quality standards are concerned. Patients using an answering service will have no feed-back as to when or if the GP will be attending, unless the GP chooses to contact them. This may be felt to be inappropriate by a GP who knows that he will call within the next 2–3 hours. This is a quality issue that must be addressed within patients' charters. In addition, if there is no telephone in the house and initial contact cannot be made by phone, a house call may have to be made, as initial contact within the charter time, even when this is not clinically appropriate.

Design of out-of-hours provision

The provision of out-of-hours service is part of the 24-hour commitment that each GP makes in signing a contract with the FHSA. It is therefore up to each GP to ensure that the care provided for patients between the hours of 7.00 pm and 7.00 am weekdays and from 12 noon Saturday until 7.00 am Monday is of a satisfactory standard.

Financial implications

Out-of-hours can be split into two categories:

- that which merely fulfils part of general medical service
- that between the hours of 10.00 pm and 8.00 am which attracts an item of service fee.

It is important in business planning terms that the responsibility of each partner in respect of calls that arrive between these hours is clear.

It is not mandatory within the terms of service for GPs to visit patients who request a call, and each individual GP decides whether or not a visit is warranted. Every practitioner is aware of patients who generally ring for advice and do not specifically request the GP to visit. If the call is received between 10.00 pm and 8.00 am, however, there is an opportunity cost if a partner does not make a visit. In other words, it would have been possible for that GP to have earned the higher rate fee for the practice but made the decision not to do so.

This can obviously be inequitable if one GP meets all requests for visits received during the hours of eligibility while another GP does none. This can be dealt with in different ways, for example:

- by having guidelines on the sort of calls that require visits and those where contact with the patient by telephone is deemed to be reasonable and acceptable to the practice
- by having the income generated by night visits allocated to each partner.

In the example cited above, if one GP received requests for and made 100 night visits then he would receive £4615 at 1993 rates, whereas the other GP who received 100 calls but made no visits would receive nothing.

The financial implications must also be considered of using either cooperatives (if the cooperative is deemed to be eligible for the lower rate fee, the opportunity of earning the higher fee is lost) or deputizing services (where not only is income lost but the service also costs). It is also important to know when the night visits are made. For example, it may be acceptable to GPs to make calls before midnight and thus be eligible personally for their higher rate fees, but to use a deputizing locum or cooperative service after midnight, thus ensuring a full night's sleep in return for the actual and opportunity cost that this entails. It is important in the modelling process that the percentage of practice income for each

GP that a decision such as this represents is calculated, so that a full view of the impact of the decision on the profit share at the end of the year is obtained.

There is no correct solution for the provision of out-of-hours contact, and the business planning approach is to lay out a number of possible scenarios to allow the practice partners to judge what suits them at the present time.

Consultation

Detailed planning has now succeeded in bringing the GP and the patient together. Consultation is the basic process of general practice. Stott and Davis[1] described a framework for analysing each consultation with a patient, which consists of four areas:

- area A: presenting complaint
- area B: modification of help-seeking behaviour
- area C: continuing care
- area D: identifying risk factors.

This framework can be used in a planning sense. The GP can examine the patient's record before the consultation and can determine what activity is required in area C (review of any existing on-going medical conditions, eg hypertension, hypothyroidism) and area D (any risk factors that are not recorded, eg blood pressure, cervical smear status).

What the patient says to the GP during the consultation (area A) and the context/stage of the illness that is presented (area B) will determine whether the GP follows up the plan that had been devised before the consultation started. This model shows one way in which a management plan can be determined.

Diagnostic investigations

GPs appear to fall into two camps:

- those who make a diagnosis rapidly and then collect information in order to support it
- those who need to collect information and collate it in order to reach a diagnosis.

The whole purpose of investigating patients must be clarified before decisions can be made about its usefulness. If investigations are to be ordered, it is important that the GP is clear as to what impact the result of the investigation will have on the management of the patient. The use of routine investigations is to be discouraged.

Open access

- What is the meaning of open access to investigations?
- What is the implication of such open access?

Open access can be regarded as direct referral to 'second-level specialists', eg radiologists and pathologists, rather than having to refer to 'first-level specialists', eg physicians and surgeons. The GP using such a service must be aware of:

- whether the test is accurate
- the false-positive and false-negative rates
- whether the test is appropriate; in other words, can it answer the question that is being posed by the GP in order to strengthen the hypothesis about the patient's condition?
- the impact of the 'result/answer' on the management plan for the patient.

It may be wiser to outline the clinical situation and indicate the question that requires an answer rather than to specify the exact investigation required.

For example, a consultant radiologist may have clearer ideas than a GP of the most cost-effective investigation to answer the question that has been posed. If a patient presents with clinical symptoms of a torn knee cartilage, it makes more sense to order magnetic resonance imaging as the first investigation rather than obtaining an unnecessary and wasteful plain radiograph first.

Guidelines

The development of practice guidelines has become so popular that some people speak of standard mania[2]. Although the establishment of such guidelines can undoubtedly be extremely useful, a note of caution needs to be sounded – the appropriate method for developing valid and reliable guidelines has not yet been established. There is a great deal of difference between deciding on and writing guidelines and achieving their implementation within the practice.

Prescribing

One definition of coarseness is that which happens in real life rather than that which happens in text books (*see* Chapter 5). The authors' definition of a coarse GP was 'one who decides what to treat the patient with and then makes the diagnosis fit' (*see* Chapter 5, page 52). A good example is that of a patient who presents with a red, inflamed throat. If the GP decides that this patient is ill and toxic, a decision may be made that it will be to the patient's benefit to receive penicillin. If the GP wishes such a patient to receive penicillin, he will record a diagnosis of tonsillitis, thereby justifying the choice of this drug. If the GP does not feel that the patient is particularly ill, however, a diagnosis of pharyngitis may be recorded. This does not justify the use of penicillin, and the GP will recommend simple home remedies including gargles and paracetamol.

The downward pressures on prescribing are formidable at present and show no signs of abating. It is within this climate that much of the planning activity takes place: whether the practice likes it or not, costs need to be contained. Given this, the planning required for the management of prescribing within the practice is a complex affair. Many parameters may impinge on the individual GPs when and if a prescription is written.

It is necessary to break the prescribing habits of a practice down into manageable sections to see whether change can be achieved. Planning in this sense has to be based on an audit mechanism, of which the best known is PACT (Prescribing Analysis and CosT) data. Computer systems may also provide the practice with information about which drugs are in their top 10 or top 50 prescribed (by both volume and cost) and have the advantage of being more current than the historical data provided by PACT. Ownership of prescribing may present some problems. It may be difficult to determine not only who started the prescribing habits but also who is in charge of them. If this is so, then no-one may take actual responsibility for determining whether the prescribing habits are still rational.

Audits of repeat prescribing have suggested that many of the top 20 drugs, in terms of cost, are prescribed on repeat as well as acute bases. If this is so, repeat prescribing in the practice may require attention if prescribing costs are to be managed. This will be important if the practice is:

- a high-cost/low-volume presciber
- a high-volume/low-cost prescriber

- out of line with the rest of the practices in the FHSA in any given therapeutic area, in terms of cost and volume or the most expensive and most widely used drugs.

This last is particularly important because it is in these areas that the changes (if any) will need to take place.

Some ways of reducing prescribing costs are shown in Box 7.4. Whatever system is adopted, the partners will have to decide whether they are prepared to:

- not prescribe certain drugs; this may mean an alteration in clinical practice, perhaps even a move away from best practice
- switch to generic/alternative prescribing; this may need explanation to patients
- make the changes merely prospective ie as patients are seen acutely on an individual basis, or by wider notification to patients of an alteration to established medication.

Prospective changes means that the GP has to be continually aware and alert during the consultation to alter the prescribing pattern. Retrospective changes may be achieved by a find and replace system (either manual or computer-driven). In other words, the patients are informed collectively that the practice has taken the decision to discontinue prescribing drug X in favour of drug Y. The actual mechanism is 'find, stop and commence'. Practices using computers should ensure that the software

---

Box 7.4 Ways of reducing prescribing costs

- Black list: in this system the government decides that certain drugs may not be prescribed within the NHS. There is no choice in this matter, and many drugs on this list cannot in future contribute to clinicians' expenditure. This system may also be adopted by the practice, but the method is harder to follow if the drugs are still available for prescription

- Formulary: in this system drugs are positively included for prescription. Drugs outside the list may require special procedures in order for their prescribing to take place, eg only partners are allowed to prescribe them

- Find and replace: in this system a process similar to that used in word processing is used. An identifier drug(s) is located and replaced by a cheaper alternative, which may be generic or manufactured by a specific company

exists to do this precise task. More 'find and replace' by computer methods is unacceptable, especially to defence bodies, if the *historic* record of prescribing is also altered.

Outcome measures

It is necessary to know the outcome of the consultation in order to judge whether it has been productive. There are two major parameters by which the outcome of a consultation can be judged.

* Is the patient satisfied? This is notoriously difficult to measure. It is not necessarily clear why the patient has attended. The provision of a prescription to the patient does not necessarily indicate a successful outcome. It is, of course, possible to ask – a consumer survey.

* Has there been an outcome in terms of benefit to the patient's health?

The second of these can be broken down into a number of more easily determined parameters (Box 7.5).

Box 7.5   Determination of outcome in terms of benefit to patients' health

* In terms of area A in the Stott-Davis model (*see* page 81), has the presenting complaint been dealt with adequately (either having been treated or explained)?

* Have chronic diseases been properly checked or reviewed, and have the correct guidelines and procedures been followed in dealing with these?

* Have health promotion opportunities been taken?

* Has a prescription been given? If so, is it appropriate to the needs of the patient? Does it conform to the guidelines that exist for the patient's condition within the practice?

* Has a referral been made or have investigations been ordered? If so, are these reasonable? Do they help in either elucidating the diagnosis or improving the patient's well-being or health?

* Has the GP used the other resources that are available within the practice? If a smear is required, was that done by the GP or was it delegated to another capable member of staff, eg the practice nurse?

Consultations can also be judged in business planning terms, to determine whether the full opportunity has been taken of maximizing the income that is available within the current system. This relates to items of service, targets for cytology and immunizations, and health promotion bandings. The resourcing of the practice and its subsequent earning potential lie within the hands of the partners. Many GPs talk of their practice as though it were a separate entity from themselves – a body that employs them and provides a monthly salary cheque, but over which they have no control. This, of course, is absolute nonsense. The practice is what the partners make it, and again this makes it clear that it is vital that the partners have a clear view of the outcome measures that they require.

Health gain

Health gain is being promoted by a DoH initiative[3] as an outcome measure for episodes of care, and this provides a unique opportunity to educate both GPs and consultants in creating joint guidelines in management. Health gain is a concept that can be applied to many areas of clinical work.

In Wales, the current emphasis is on the ten health gain areas shown in Box 7.6[4]. Within each of these areas, a protocol that sets out targets for the NHS has been devised. For example, the *Protocol for investment in health gain for respiratory diseases* notes the following.

Box 7.6   The ten health gain areas for Wales

- Injuries

- Learning difficulties

- Emotional health and relationships

- Respiratory diseases

- Maternal and early child health

- Cancers

- Cardiovascular disease

- Mental distress and illness

- Physical disability and discomfort

- Healthy living

- Identifiable annual expenditure on formal health services for the people of Wales related to respiratory diseases is approximately £100 million. Most of the cost is attributable to hospital care, though a considerable amount is spent on drugs in the community.

- Although quality of life is difficult to measure, real efforts to improve it, where possible, must rank high among NHS priorities.

Health gain targets

Continuing the example of respiratory diseases the original targets set included:

- The number of acute admissions to hospital for people with asthma should be reduced by the year 2002.

- Local medical committees in conjunction with local hospital consultants and directors of public health should develop standard protocols for diagnosis and treatment of respiratory diseases based on national guidelines and local circumstance by 1993.

- By 1993 local medical audit advisory groups should be encouraged through the Welsh Advisory Group on Medical Audit to consider facilitating establishment of arrangements for monitoring activity in their health care areas through clinical audit, including establishment of a database of activity providing validated comparisons over time, across areas and within practices, and improving the competence of people to manage minor self-limiting illnesses.

- Annual deaths from asthma among those aged below 45 years should be reduced by 75% by 2002.

- Compared with 1994 the proportion of people under 65 years of age with asthma who report activity limitations should be reduced by 20% by 1997 and by 50% by 2002.

A service target was set to raise to 80% the proportion of patients with perennial asthma who are in possession of a peak flow meter and a written management plan by 1997.

The mechanisms that are in place to audit whether targets have been met and whether targets can be modified in the light of new information are less clear at this juncture. An example would be the concept that self-management plans should be targeted only at those with severe asthma[5,6]. This is not easily reconciled with a target of 80% of patients with asthma having a written plan by 1997.

Impact on general practice

In the light of these comments, what impact does the concept of health gain have on the practice? The amount of glossy literature that emanates from Government shows no sign of abating. The inputs that are received by the district health commissioners will eventually be converted into a health plan for the district, which will give the purchasing intentions for the forthcoming years. Increasingly, these purchasing intentions will be couched in terms of health gain, and also be related to the strategic intention and direction (in Wales; *see* page 86).

All practices can influence the health gain targets, via the local medical committee and FHSA and directly. All practices are responsible for the management of patients, and it is the sum of this care that is expressed as health gain. It is increasingly the responsibility of the practice to translate the aspirations of the health/business plan into intentions (including purchasing intentions for fund holders) that will allow the plan to come to fruition. The practice can remain independent by ensuring that the methods chosen to achieve the various health gain targets are the sole responsibility of the practice. The practice should therefore ensure that it is judged, not by structure or methods, but by outcome.

The only caveat to this scenario is that the practice should ensure that it starts from a position comparable with the average for the district. There are social biases in any of the health gain targets. It should be remembered that the targets set by the district are an average for all of the district. If, for example, the practice is recognized as serving a socioeconomic class IV/V population, the baseline for any of the chosen parameters will be lower than the district average. In these instances the practice should not set itself an impossible task by attempting to reach the district average. Rather, it should set itself a realistic target which, though below the district average, will nevertheless contribute to the overall increase for the district.

Referral

The move towards joint guidelines between primary and secondary care for patients is often linked to the transfer of services that were previously delivered in a hospital setting to a general practice setting/premises. It is important to look at the current processes and their purpose before proposing any changes.

Processes

Referral

The GP decides that the patient needs to see a consultant:

- for an opinion/reassurance, eg in fibroadenotic breast disease, when the patient only needs to be seen once before returning to the GP

- for investigations: these may be done when the patient sees the consultant, eg sigmoidoscopy, or may need to be arranged with a further specialist

- for technical skills: these may be used when the patient sees the consultant, eg aspirating a breast cyst, or on an in-patient basis for surgical techniques. For very discrete procedures, eg removal of an in-growing toenail, an initial appointment with the consultant may not be required and the patient can be placed immediately onto the in-patient/day case waiting list.

The purpose of the referral letter is to:

- outline the current situation, together with all appropriate background information

- indicate the purpose of the referral, ie what the GP is requesting the consultant to do

- request an appointment with the consultant at the out-patient department.

Once the initial consultation has taken place, the following may occur:

Investigations

These are done by the consultant to support the hypothesis/management plan that is being formulated.

Out-patient appointment

This is used to provide information to the patient about the investigations.

Out-patient appointment after in-patient procedure

This is used to provide information to the patient about the operative procedure. It is also used to check the healing process, and possibly to end the episode by declaring the patient fit to return to a normal lifestyle.

Discharge to GP

Following an out-patient appointment, responsibility for all care is transferred back to the GP. Information about the episode and prognosis is also transferred by letter. This is almost invariably unidirectional, ie from consultant to GP, even though the patient may require life-long care and may develop other medical conditions.

Out-patient appointment (ongoing)

This is used to monitor the progress of a disease. Information about the disease and prognosis is transferred by letter.

The strategic direction for changes in the referral process can be summarized as follows.

- Health gain focused: to add years to life through a reduction in premature death, and life to years by improving well-being for both patients and the population at large.

- People-centred: should value people as individuals and manage services to this end.

- Resource-effective: should strive to achieve the most cost-effective balance in its use of available resources.

With these strategic principles in mind, the referral process can be changed as discussed.

8 | Planning for Fundholding Status

Considerable documentation is available to explain the theory of fundholding[1], and this should be consulted for more detailed guidance on fundholding issues. Basically, GPs who meet certain list size and other criteria have a delegated fund in respect of:

- hospital and community health services
- prescribing
- directly employed staff.

Once the practice accepts the fund, the GPs choose how to allocate the fund between these three elements. This section outlines some of the practical issues relevant to fundholding.

Commencing fundholding

When a practice is approved to be a fundholder, it takes on new responsibilities, as detailed in Box 8.1. Given these responsibilities and taking into account the practice's relationship with the RHA/DHA/FHSA, some realistic objectives for the first year may include:

- surviving year 1 relatively unscathed
- obtaining a 'better' level of care for practice patients than was previously possible, eg on-site physiotherapy
- deriving mutually agreed, detailed waiting lists with provider hospitals
- assessing practice clinical records to determine what morbidity data can be contributed to health planning

---

Box 8.1   Responsibilities of a fundholding practice

- Purchasing specified health services
- Health planning
- Stewardship of public funds
- Provision of certified accounts
- Public accountability for its actions
- Regular reporting on finance and activity to the FHSA
- Negotiation of service agreements in respect of patients
- Monitoring of the performance of hospital providers and its own fund
- Ensuring the accuracy of data entered onto the GP fundholding computer system

---

- reducing overall prescribing costs by x% or increasing generic prescribing to y% of the total.

Practice profile

Assessment of health needs is vital for the effective deployment of health service resources. Fundholding practices have had their funds set on a historical basis to date, but the DoH is proposing to introduce a weighted capitation basis in the future. This is intended to avoid the inequities that are implicit in a historical funding basis. The whole concept of health needs assessment can seem quite overwhelming, and it is worth discussing local approaches with the director of public health medicine at the DHA.

All purchasers, GP fundholders and DHAs will be expected to demonstrate that their health plans and purchasing strategies are focused towards attaining health gain for their respective populations. In order to do this, needs assessment is mandatory. An incrementalist approach is recommended, in which the data currently held are examined to see whether they provide meaningful direct or proxy measures of health status. The data can then be interpreted in the light of relevant factors, such as:

- epidemiology
- morbidity

- mortality
- census data
- demography
- clinical (primary and secondary) care audit.

Fundholders will be joint, even if minority, commissioners of health services with their DHA. In the coming years, commissioners will be expected to demonstrate how their joint strategy is achieving outcomes. This will require commissioners to:

- assess the health needs of their population
- rank them by priority
- deploy the limited resources available.

In this way the health needs of the population can be effectively targeted.

Preparatory year fee

A preparatory year fee is available to practices who wish to become fundholders and have received RHA/FHSA approval to commence the preparatory (data collection) year. The fee is designed to meet the costs associated with the preparatory year tasks. Relevant approved expenditure may be reimbursed up to a maximum of £17,500 (1993/94). Practices are required to submit a plan to their FHSA outlining their expenditure profile. The allowance may be used for various items including:

- employing staff for data collection activities
- training practice staff in fundholding procedures/software
- paying for locum cover while GPs are actively involved in the data collection period
- obtaining specialist advice relating to financial management or negotiation
- purchasing relevant equipment including computers.

The fee is normally reimbursed to the practice monthly in arrears as expenditure occurs. The FHSA usually asks for a spending/action plan (or business plan, as the terms are used interchangeably) that specifies:

- how the preparatory year fee will be spent

- the reimbursement that will be sought in respect of computerization for fundholding
- how the data collection action will be structured, monitored and completed
- proposals for the future management of fundholding activity.

Management allowance

Once a practice has been approved as a fundholder, it is entitled to an annual management allowance, subject to a maximum reimbursement (of £35,000 in 1993/94), to permit the practice to manage its fund effectively. This may be used for:

- wages or salaries of a fund manager and/or information officer
- payment for a locum to allow one of the practice GPs to become involved in the clinical aspects of service agreements and health planning
- office equipment
- training, both initial and ongoing, together with attendance at seminars and conferences regarding fundholding.

As with the preparatory year fee, the practice is required annually to submit a spending plan to the FHSA. This is normally reimbursed 1 month in arrears, given proof of expenditure.

Computer system

In order to gain fundholding status, practices have to demonstrate that they have (or will have) the capability to operate the fundholding software. This software is available from a number of authorized suppliers who have conformed to the DoH specifications. Depending on the practice's current level of computerization, it is possible to operate the software either as an integrated system or as a stand-alone system. Issues to consider include:

- the availability of terminals in consulting rooms
- the capability of the processing unit (model, speed, RAM, hard disk capacity, operating system)
- requirements for linking branch surgeries (land line, modem)

- current software supplier package and the possibility of full clinical integration.

Whenever possible, it is recommended that practices purchase a fund-holding system that can be integrated with the clinical system. The FHSA is usually able to advise practices on their choice of software. Practices should buy and install the system in sufficient time for staff to become familiar with the package before fundholding becomes operational. The FHSA will be able to confirm the current arrangements for reimbursement.

The fundholding software has been written specifically to meet the DoH specifications. It is principally an accounts system that supports the double-entry bookkeeping standards used throughout the GP fundholding accounts. The system effectively operates as a referrals ledger and a nominal ledger to record the following processes:

- accounting transactions

- invoice receipt and payment

- monitoring costs of individual patients and identification of high-cost patients

- referrals to secondary services

- producing predefined reports on referral and financial activity by the practice.

Data collection process

During the preparatory year, prospective fundholding practices are required to collect data relating to a specific period in order to build a complete record of chargeable usage. The data are based on the discharge letters that come into the practice from hospitals, together with requests for diagnostic tests and direct access services. The absence of a weighted capitation formula or detailed practice-level information from provider units means that the practice records themselves are the only reliable source of data on which to assess the use that a practice has made of hospital services in previous years.

Probably the best way to undertake the task is to use experienced practice staff whose previous knowledge of the practice's organization and records system will:

- ensure confidentiality

- enable them to cope with more complex aspects

- facilitate efficient completion of the exercise.

The practice may wish to employ temporary staff to release permanent staff to undertake the data collection or make overtime payments to existing staff to undertake the task out of surgery hours.

An essential prerequisite for successful completion of the data collection is the appointment of a partner to oversee the operation. This appointment will:

- provide the necessary clinical interpretation

- ensure the accuracy of the data collected

- permit a system of internal quality control to be introduced as data extraction progresses.

Small batches of notes and completed forms should be abstracted at random and assessed by the partner supervising the data extraction to identify problems before it is too late to rectify them.

Data collection is the essential first step in calculating the hospital services element of the fund. The FHSA, RHA and DHA will each have a role in ensuring that the exercise is carried out accurately and in accordance with DoH guidelines. The FHSA provides a first point of contact for advice regarding interpretation of the methodology, while the DHA should be involved in the exercise from the outset so that it can be satisfied with the overall conduct of the data collection.

After collection the data are validated by the practice's host DHA and RHA. As these data form the basis of the fund calculation, it cannot be overemphasized how important it is to get this right. Practices will need to collect data in respect of:

- specific elective surgical procedures

- out-patient attendances

- consultant domiciliary visits

- diagnostic tests (pathology, radiology)

- direct access services (physiotherapy, speech therapy, chiropody, dietetics, occupational therapy)

- community nursing services (district nursing, health visiting).

The RHA or FHSA will provide the practice with either standard forms or a computer program, so that data can be collected in a standardized format. Many practices will hold good-quality referral data on manual or computerized records, because they are already required to collect information for annual reports to the FHSA.

The process for determining the hospital services element is as follows.

- Practices collect data on their referral patterns for hospital services that are included in the fund.

- In order to ensure the accuracy of the data, the RHA reconciles the data collected by the practice with data obtained from provider units (where available).

- Any significant changes in anticipated list size are taken into account.

- The hospital services value is calculated on the basis of the agreed data and price tariffs from those providers from whom the service is currently received.

The agreed level of service at the end of the exercise forms essential data for the practice to determine the need for contracts. The volumes of services will assist in deciding the types of contract to be used. The data will also indicate where these services have been obtained historically. Practices do not need to wait for costings to be applied to the level of service before starting contract negotiations. Where practices contract within their past referral patterns, they normally have assurance that prices charged will be consistent with the prices used in the costing of the agreed level of service. The RHA is the final arbiter in cases of dispute about the level of service to be funded and the allocation necessary to fund the agreed level of service.

The FHSA will provide the practice with a sample of patients from which data will be collected. This sample will be based on the current practice list and will comprise either 50% of patients or a minimum of 6000 patients, whichever is the greater. Practices are encouraged to work on a 100% sample. The patient sample will be produced at random by the FHSA, but practices should discuss their requirements with the FHSA to ensure that the list is provided on the same basis on which the practice records are organized, eg by surgery, GP, or sex.

The hospital services element of the fund is based around three basic principles.

- The fund covers patients permanently on the fundholder's list.

- The fund covers those treatments and procedures on the list of approved goods and services.

- The fundholder is only financially responsible for activity that has been initiated or authorized by the fundholding practice.

The practice should take all reasonable steps to avoid underreporting, and the following points are worth considering.

- The whole of a patient's case notes should be accessed, as summaries of the practice's notes and hospital discharge summaries can be misleading.

- Written confirmation of treatments received, eg discharge summaries, may sometimes take weeks or months to arrive and are often filed separately from the part of the notes that covers the relevant 2-year period.

- It is important to check whether any chargeable procedures have been undertaken following non-chargeable in-patient episodes.

- Patients may have been referred to a chargeable paramedical service following a consultant attendance, eg to physiotherapy by a consultant orthopaedic surgeon.

- Where a consultant is known to never or very seldom send discharge summaries, the practice may have to collect data from the consultant's secretary at the hospital.

- Evidence of tertiary referrals by consultants must be sought.

- In-patient or day case activity may consist of multiple procedures or investigations at a single attendance. These should be disaggregated and recorded separately.

- Considerable detective work may be needed when trying to reconstruct what happened to a patient from inadequate data.

The information collected is aggregated to obtain summary activity levels for budget-setting purposes. These summary data are sent to the RHA who will check, for example, the completeness of the data, the validity of the codes used and the number of emergency in-patient and day case episodes. The RHA will report its findings to the practice for corrections and, after revalidation, will send a draft summary report to the DHA. This will be the basis for agreeing the outcome of the data collection exercise. The DHA will then use its data sources, collected from hospital systems, to check whether the activity levels of the data collection seem reasonable.

When the practice, RHA, FHSA and DHA have agreed on the summary activity, a final report of the data is produced and grossed up to create an agreed level of activity, reflecting the whole practice list. This report will be used by the DHA for costing the activity and placing a value on the fund.

Changes during the fundholding year, eg significant growth in practice list size or new patients on high-cost drugs, should be monitored and reported back to the FHSA/RHA so that the value of the overall fund may be periodically reviewed for adequacy.

Staffing requirements

The availability of a suitable management resource is critical to success in fundholding. This may be already available within the team or may be provided by arrangement with the FHSA. If not, then consideration must be given to recruiting a suitably qualified person. This is a key partner activity, and it can be costly to the practice in both financial and human terms to make selection mistakes. The purpose of the selection procedure is to predict the future job performance of each of the candidates in order to select the right person for the job. In order to achieve some predictive validity from the exercise, it is necessary to have some objective criteria in the form of:

- a detailed job description
- a person specification.

An example of each document for a fund manager's post is given in Appendix F, together with a job description for an information officer. The job description and person specification can only be constructed once the partners/lead GP have determined the relationship they require with the new manager and the level of *delegation* that is appropriate.

Delegation

Delegation may be defined as giving others the authority to act on your behalf, accompanying it with responsibility and accountability for results. It thus involves:

- authority: the right to make decisions, take actions and give orders
- responsibility: the job and/or tasks the employee is given to do
- accountability: the employee's liability to the partnership and the obligation to accept responsibility and use authority.

The advantages of delegation are shown in Box 8.2.
The GP should delegate when:

- there is more work than can be effectively carried out alone
- it is not possible to allow sufficient time for priority tasks
- there is a need to develop a member of staff
- the job can be done adequately by an employee.

Once the partnership has decided to delegate specific managerial/fund-holding matters, both parties need to understand:

Box 8.2   Advantages of delegation

- It relieves GPs of routine and less critical tasks and frees them for more important work – clinical practice, planning, organizing, motivating and controlling

- It extends the capacity to manage

- It reduces delay in decision-making, provided that authority is delegated close to the point of action

- It allows decisions to be taken at the level where the details are known

- It develops the capacity of subordinates to make decisions, get things done and take responsibility

---

- what the staff are expected to do
- the authority devolved to make decisions
- the problems/issues that must be referred back
- progress or completion reports that must be submitted and the timescale involved
- the basis for monitoring progress
- the resources and help available to get the work done.

The type of work that the GP should delegate includes routine and operational matters, jobs that a manager can do as well or better than a GP can, and jobs that require the specialized skill of a manager. When examining the potential for successful delegation of management of the practice fund, it is worth thinking about how the process will work. Having considered the basis for decision-making in the practice and allowing for partner interactions, thought should be given to the allocation of responsibility between partners and the interactions between partners, manager and staff. Therefore, an analysis of available resources should be undertaken to provide:

- an agreed statement of expertise, abilities and role preferences of individual partners

- an estimate of activity time, analysed between different practice activities and including the expected demands of fundholding

- development of goal statements by individual partners.

Appointing a fundholding manager

Having determined the nature of the job, the kind of person required and the working relationship involved, a short list of candidates for interview can be drawn up from the applicants.

Interview is probably the most commonly used form of selection. It is relatively quick, easy and cheap. It is unreliable, however, as a method of predicting job performance, as the interview lacks objectivity. Sources of bias stem from the interviewers, the practice and the candidates themselves.

- Interviewers may lack skills in interviewing or may be unclear about the knowledge and skills that the job requires.

- Interviewers may have preconceptions and stereotypical views, which they project onto the candidate.

- There is a tendency for interviewers to select in their 'own image', and they may choose a candidate they like rather than one who has the ability to do the job.

- The practice, ie the partners jointly, may fail to provide job descriptions and person specifications (as discussed earlier) or other clear selection criteria for recruiters.

- The selection procedures may be inadequate, and the practice may not have provided the recruiters with adequate training.

- There may be a lack of monitoring by and accountability to the partnership for selection decisions taken by individual partners.

- Unrealistic time pressures may result in inadequate preparation and too little time and attention being given to the selection process.

- Finally, candidates may be unprepared or they may expect to fail because of similar past experiences.

Some examples of interview questions that allow recruiters to thoroughly test candidates are included in Appendix G. Supplementary selection techniques include observation of group tasks, personality profiling and team role analysis.

Building relationships

It is useful to consider the roles of the practice's partners in fundholding. These include:

- the RHA
- the FHSA
- the DHA
- NHS trusts
- directly managed units.

The RHA has overall responsibility for the effective operation of the fundholding scheme, and its functions in this role are shown in Box 8.3. In some regions, and in Wales where there is no RHA, much of this role has been delegated to the FHSAs.

The FHSAs continue to exercise their current responsibilities in relation to all GPs for delivery of health care with respect to general medical services. In addition, they have new responsibilities in relation to fundholding, as shown in Box 8.4.

The DHA and fundholding practices have no direct relationship with one another, but both are searching for high-quality and cost-effective health care for their respective populations. GP fundholding covers only a limited range of services, and the DHA remains responsible for purchasing health care services outside the scope of the fund which are provided to the practice's patients. As joint purchasers/commissioners of health care, it is worth examining common interests in relation to particular providers, eg quality and innovative methods of service delivery. Practices should advise their DHA when patients approach or exceed the £6000 threshold for hospital services in the fund, above which the DHA is liable to pay for treatment.

Box 8.3 Functions of the RHA in fundholding

- Assessment of practice suitability for fundholding status
- Conciliation in contractual disputes
- Determination of the value of the fund
- Approval of expenditure for the preparatory year fee and management allowance
- Source of advice and guidance to fundholders in their purchasing role

---

Box 8.4   Responsibilities of the FHSA in fundholding

- Holding fundholders' budgets and paying invoices on their behalf

- Responsibility for routine monitoring of fundholder expenditure. Each practice is required to submit each month a number of reports covering expenditure and activity to the FHSA. The FHSA submits a summary of these reports to the RHA

- Advising the RHA on the practice's initial and continuing suitability for fundholding status

- Calculating the staff and prescribing elements of the fund

- Validation of the preparatory year fee and management allowance expenditure, and reimbursement to fundholders for relevant computer costs

---

Negotiation

Negotiation is an important element in the establishment of relationships, particularly those of the practice with its providers. There is a need to establish trust when the negotiating relationships are considered. These form the basis for suitable long-term purchaser/provider relationships and encourage adherence to quality standards with emphasis being placed on improving services/products. Factors that may influence the relationship include:

- the level of advance preparation

- the interpersonal skills of the negotiators

- a lack of understanding of the other party's interests

- short-term perspectives as opposed to long-term objectives

- the reasonableness of the changes sought

- awareness of the limitations applied to the negotiations.

Negotiation skills

The way in which the negotiating team is constructed plays an important part in the success of all negotiations. The GP and manager may negotiate as a team, where they act as the practice representatives. Because the process of negotiation is quite complex, it is suggested that the practice has a negotiating team, which might be as small as two people or possibly as large as four. Once it gets beyond this number it is difficult to manage, and some team members will appear to take no part in the negotiation. The actual negotiations often occur between only one or two individuals while others look on, and this is not a very efficient use of people's time.

It is useful for one team member to act as the devil's advocate when planning negotiations. This will indicate potential weaknesses in the practice's arguments and develop a strong commitment to the practice view. Sometimes negotiating teams develop a cosy atmosphere and become unwilling to discuss the potential weaknesses of their arguments, fearing that this may upset other team colleagues. This has been called 'group think'. By legitimizing the role of devil's advocate, group think is avoided.

Another valuable feature of having more than one person involved in negotiations is that different styles can be used. At a simple level this could be the manager taking a hard line, while the GP takes a much softer line.

Representatives obviously want to do well on behalf of the practice in any negotiation meeting they attend, and there is a powerful desire to succeed. It can be disastrous, however, to go into a negotiation without being fully briefed. Quite often quick wits will suffice, but there will be times when a reluctance to admit incomplete knowledge might produce some embarrassing results for the practice. Some key issues worthy of consideration include:

- do we know what negotiation *means*?

- do we know *when* we are negotiating?

- do we know *how* to negotiate?

- do *they* know how to negotiate?

- do we acknowledge our own negotiating *strengths* and *weaknesses*?

The principles of successful negotiation are shown in Box 8.5.

Feedback in negotiations

It is essential that any presentation is listened to and observed carefully. To be of value, feedback should:

- be based on observed behaviour, not the individual's personality traits, though emotional reactions to different stages of the presentation of the case should be considered

- provide examples of why what the negotiator is proposing seems impractical, rather than simply saying that it cannot be done

- share ideas and give information, without necessarily giving advice.

Box 8.5   Some negotiating principles[2]

- Do not negotiate if you do not have to
- Be prepared
- Let the other side do the work
- Apply power gently
- Make the other side compete
- Leave yourself some room
- Maintain integrity (long-term credibility)
- Listen, do not talk
- Maintain eye contact
- Allow time for the other side to accustom to your ideas

Each stage of a negotiation is about exploring the alternatives, not always providing an answer. Negotiators should be positive and identify at least one strength as well as areas needing improvement in their opponent's proposals, and seek commitment to develop any weaknesses. A questioning approach should be used to enable the presenter to identify his own weaknesses.

Negotiating styles

These are extremely important.

- A *win–lose* style is competitive and quite tough on all of the participants. It leads to an adversarial climate and entrenched views.
- A *win–win* style is collaborative and derives mutual benefits through a climate of cooperation, thus encouraging openness, truthfulness and greater involvement.

Skilled negotiators have a clear sense of direction which produces fewer counter-proposals and requires the use of fewer 'defending' or 'attacking' comments. They give reasoned explanations leading to any statement of disagreement, rather than the other way round. They spend considerable time seeking information and invest time in testing and understanding their opponents' position, summarizing progress and being confident enough to 'express' feelings.

Conflict

Inevitably, some negotiations will not go as well as anticipated, and this can lead to conflict. It is therefore worth realizing that conflict can be positive when it:

- helps to open up discussion of an issue
- results in problems being solved
- increases the level of individual involvement and interest in an issue
- improves communication
- releases stored emotions
- helps people to develop their abilities.

Conflict can be negative, however, when it:

- diverts people from dealing with the important issues
- creates feelings of dissatisfaction among the people involved
- leads to individuals and groups becoming isolated and uncooperative.

The symptoms of conflict within and between groups include:

- poor communications (horizontally and vertically)
- intergroup hostility and jealousy
- interpersonal friction
- escalation to arbitration
- proliferation of rules and regulations, norms and myths.

There is often low morale due to frustration at inefficiency.

The causes of conflict are often competing objectives and ideologies, or concerns about territory or spheres of influence. Friction between objectives and ideologies leading to conflict can arise when formal objectives overlap or concealed objectives exist. This may also occur when the contractual relationship is unclear. In medicine in particular, clinicians are conscious of their status and this can lead to conflict when territorial violation occurs – and GP fundholding is changing the nature of the GP/consultant relationship.

The tactics employed by negotiators are often similar to the symptoms and are commonly the seeds of further conflict, but are not the root cause. They include:

- information control (information gives power)

- information distortion (misuse of information control)
- rules and regulations used as both defensive and offensive mechanisms
- information channels (the response to rules and regulations is often the 'informal network')
- denigration or tale-telling, to identify flaws in opponents.

Such tactics often lead to the hardening of conflict, with distortion and control of information. What commenced as collaboration degenerates into hard bargaining and the misapplication of individual and group energies.

The purpose of a practice response strategy is to turn conflict into fruitful competition or purposeful argument. If this is not possible, the aim should be to control it, or ultimately, to make a positive decision to ignore it. Fruitful competition can be achieved by:

- agreement on a common goal or objective
- making all the information available to participants
- developing appropriate coordination mechanisms
- establishing a communication system that creates trust
- ensuring that considerations of role and territory do not conflict with the overall goal.

Control of conflict strategies may include:

- resorting to arbitration (but beware of a spiral effect)
- developing acceptable rules and procedures
- coordinating devices, eg as the creation of a new body to deal with the problem.

Other options include confrontation, separation, or avoidance.

Making meetings productive

Every meeting attended has an opportunity cost – something else could have been done with the time. It is therefore important to:

- establish the purpose of each meeting
- clarify what the meeting is trying to achieve
- summarize the objectives of the meeting.

One key activity is planning ahead to ensure that those attending know what is to be discussed and why and to notify them in good time. In meetings dealing with contract issues, any necessary details of activity or prices should be obtained in good time. Thought should be given to the location for the meeting (are the familiar surroundings of the surgery best?) and to who will chair the meeting. The need for prior preparation cannot be overstated. It is necessary to produce a structured agenda and to allow sufficient time for discussion. It is always advisable to insist that minutes are taken. Throughout, an open mind facilitates discussion, so the chairman should listen, observe, contribute, summarize and control.

It is important to have effective follow up to the meeting, and copies of the minutes must be distributed. These should be a clear summary of events to ensure that any disagreements may be highlighted and addressed. This also provides the opportunity for review, to assess whether the objectives were achieved and if the process could be improved. The minutes should also include an action plan summarizing what is to be done, by whom and by when.

Some disruptive tactics of which the chairman should be aware are shown in Box 8.6.

Consortia

Fundholding practices may wish to cooperate and form management consortia in order to perform such activities as planning and contracting. This allows them to achieve:

Box 8.6   Disruptive tactics in meetings

- Arriving late/leaving early

- Engaging in private conversations

- Keeping talking, even when there is nothing to say

- Never volunteering for jobs, but criticizing others freely

- Rustling papers

- Falling asleep and snoring

- Repeatedly looking at watches, tapping pens, or interrupting

- Creating diversions by dropping things, passing round sandwiches, tea, etc

- Reopening discussions about topics already decided, particularly when the meeting has finished

- the advantages of greater purchasing power, thus exerting more influence over providers during the contracting process

- economies of scale

- exchange of ideas for service developments.

Alternatively, where practices do not meet the size criteria for fundholding recognition in their own right, they may combine with another practice to become a single fundholder. Most practices are of such a size that their population is a fraction of that of their host DHA, and as the fund is for limited services only, the practice's buying power is small in comparison with that of DHA/FHSA purchasers. Working with other fundholders in a management consortium allows the consortium to become a significant force for change in discussions with both hospital clinicians and managers.

On a practical level, particularly for practices combining to hold one fund, the implications of present and future accommodation requirements must be addressed, eg at which practice will staff be located, in which room(s), the requirements for office equipment and who are the ultimate owners.

The fund is a single entity distributed between combining practices who must therefore:

- have an agreement that confirms that any act by a member in relation to the fund binds the other members of the combining practices

- have an agreement relating to apportionment of the fund and policies for prescribing and contracting that are common to all of the practices

- agree on the procedures that will be followed in the event of one member overspending the fund

- be aware that the management and preparatory allowances available are limited to the same amount for combined practices as for single practices.

Service agreements

The most important step in the negotiation process is the timeliness of the opening dialogue. This should commence as soon as practical, so that all parties can quickly establish what can or cannot be achieved in the short, medium and long term. The contract or service agreement between purchasers and providers has not been tested in law for enforceability; rather it sets out the best intentions of both parties with respect to the various understandings between them.

The whole intent of the negotiation should be to build relationships so that issues are resolved in private rather than in public. Such 'trust', however, may not always be forthcoming. However expert in negotiation a GP becomes, even the most exacting quality standards will be meaningless unless they are:

- realistic
- achievable
- measurable
- specific
- few in number
- deliverable in time.

In negotiating the purchaser/provider service agreement, it is inevitable that a GP will experience a wide range of demands on him, which include:

- finding their room for manoeuvre constrained by 'bureaucratic' rules and procedures, ie the constraints of the GP fundholding scheme

- pressure from inside and outside the practice to demonstrate success that can be perceived by others

- the possibility that clinicians for each party will know and be familiar with each other. Negotiations often demand challenging arguments, which can be perceived as damaging to previous good clinical relationships.

Fundholders are able to negotiate service agreements with a number of different types of provider including NHS trusts, directly managed units, NHS laboratories, special health authorities, private clinics, hospitals and laboratories, and other providers of health care services.

Types of service agreement

Service agreements are of four types.

- Block contracts are the simplest type. The features of block contracts include the simplicity of monitoring them, the costs not being related to the resources used or work done, and their non-reliance on detailed knowledge of volume of activity.

When using block contracts, the software requires a *notional cost* for each treatment, so that the cost of hospital services for individual patients can be monitored. The notional cost is an estimate of the cost of the treatment based on the price of the block contract and the number of patients that the fundholder expects to refer under the contract. This type of contract requires the least administrative effort, but minimizes the practice's options for influencing service delivery.

- Cost and volume contracts allow the practice to have more control over the service provided and to link payment to activity. A given level of activity is negotiated at an agreed price, with a percentage margin either side (either volume or value). The concept of the threshold enables the cost and volume contract to suit many circumstances. The information requirements and administrative effort, however, are greater than those of a block contract.

- Cost per case contracts are the most administratively demanding and should be used for the most exceptional referrals to occasional providers. If a cost per case contract has been set up for several cases, the fundholding implications are the same as a cost and volume contract with a threshold of zero. Individual cost per case contracts are often referred to as extra-contractual referrals (ECRs).

- Fixed-price non-attributable contracts are similar to block contracts in as much as the overall price for the services provided is fixed. They differ, however, in that the overall costs do not have to be notionally attributed to individual patients.

The elements common to any service agreement are given in Box 8.7.

Choosing the service agreement

Having considered the relative advantages and disadvantages of the above mentioned options, it should be borne in mind that fundholders are charged with remaining within their fund allocation. When choosing from the contract types, it is important to assess how much confidence the practice has in the data collection exercise based on previous discharge/activity patterns. An inadequate assessment of activity in a cost and volume contract exposes the practice to unquantifiable financial risk. Reducing that risk by a cost per case approach carries a correspondingly significant increase in administrative effort.

Risk is inherent when practices deploy resources on the basis of incomplete and/or out-of-date information, given the practice's relative inexperience in making planning judgements and the constraints of operating within a health service bureaucracy that requires commitments within often unrealistic time-scales. The level of risk is diminished by a cooperative approach with the DHA/FHSA providers, thus allowing sharing of information, knowledge and experience.

Box 8.7   Elements of a service agreement

- *Introduction* sets out who the parties are, what the agreement is about and its status, eg block, cost and volume etc

- *Definitions* (optional) clarify the exact meaning of terms and phrases used

- *Statement of the range of services* describes what the agreement covers, in what volume, to what standards, and what monitoring processes are allowed. It specifies what data each party will provide to the other and the duration of the agreement

- *Location* sets out where the services are to be delivered

- *Standards* define the expected clinical and non-clinical quality aspects of the service

- *Price* specifies what will be paid for the specific items of service and exactly what is covered by such terms. It may also take account of variances, eg inflation, changed referral patterns

- *Terms of payment* denotes when money will change hands and specifies any penalties for late settlement

- *Arbitration* describes what will be done to reach a solution if both parties cannot agree about an aspect of the service

- *Monitoring* describes the process by which the agreement will be effectively monitored

---

Setting contracts with providers outside the NHS

While there is still some debate about the legal enforceability of service agreements within the NHS, arrangements with external bodies constitute legal contracts. Contracts may be placed with:

- private clinics or hospitals
- private laboratories
- charitable trusts
- voluntary organizations.

When considering such options, it is important to confirm that the professional staff who will be delivering the care have the necessary qualifications, training and experience. The issue of professional indemnity should also be confirmed.

Before entering into any arrangement, the practice should find out as much as possible about the company from independent sources. The practice needs to know that the company has the financial resources to meet its commitments in both the short and long term.

Service agreements within the NHS are often couched in the very broadest terms, which is clearly insufficient in a legally enforceable contract. The objectives of the contract need to be clearly stated to enable determination of whether they have been achieved. Failure to do this may involve the practice in paying for a service that it is not receiving.

GP fundholders are only permitted to contract for services for a maximum of 1 year, which may conflict with the provider's objective of medium-to-long-term revenue stability. This is particularly important if the provider has to make an initial investment in staff or facilities to deliver the contract, and it is advisable to discuss this aspect early in the negotiations.

Equity with non-fundholders

GP fundholding has been criticized for creating a two-tier health care system. When setting service agreements, fundholders need to be conscious

---

Box 8.8   Issues relevant to improving service: an example in obstetrics and gynaecology

- Number of women of child-bearing age
- Planned development in the area
- Existing resources/services
- Availability of midwives and other staff
- Extent of private care provision
- Demography/economic characteristics of the practice and its catchment population
- Trends/fashions in gynaecological care
- Neonatal/maternal mortality rates
- Availability of funds to purchase services
- Legislation
- Political climate, both medical and general
- Transport arrangements for patients
- Public opinion

of the impact of their demands on non-fundholding GPs. A carefully negotiated contract aimed at the general improvement of quality within a particular service/hospital/department is unlikely to attract criticism if it can be demonstrated that the benefits will be available to all patients.

Setting contracts for hospital services

When determining where to place service agreements for hospital services, a practice will consider issues relating to both quality and cost. Factors that affect the quality of service include:

- effectiveness: benefits and outcomes of interventions as assessed by clinical audit
- appropriateness: facilities and support services
- timeliness: time required to access the service
- accessibility: convenience for patients
- acceptability: clinical reporting to GP, patient satisfaction survey, responsive contracting arrangements and quality reporting.

Practice staff

This is probably the most straightforward element of the fund to calculate, because it is the aspect about which the practice has the best information and most control. Early discussions should be held with the FHSA, and it is important to confirm that the calculation includes an element for training and relief payments, at least to the same level as historical usage by the practice. Any proposed developments should be incorporated into the funding.

Community services

The principal constituents of community services are health visiting and district nursing, and many practices will have pertinent questions about the role of nursing middle-management. Under the new arrangements between practices and community providers, a closer working relationship within the practice (between GPs and attached staff) and with provider general management is being developed. This has implications for the size of the overheads for nursing management included in the service agreement.

Changes in service patterns

Fundholding has already begun to influence the GP/consultant relationship, and there is considerable anecdotal evidence of consultants now being more prepared to provide services that GPs request. Provider hospitals are now encouraging their clinical staff to visit GPs to discuss how services could be improved. This is certainly a good marketing tactic by the hospitals, as it more closely matches their 'products' with the GPs' 'want' and makes it less likely that the GPs will change their referral patterns.

Most practices will wish to place service agreements with local provider hospitals. In urban areas this can still leave the practice with considerable choice, while rural practices may be limited by geographical practicalities. In these circumstances, the purchaser/provider relationship is even more dependent on goodwill, the relative balance of power, influence and mutual trust. It is also likely that no financial savings may be possible from the hospital/community element where the fundholder has limited or no choice of providers. In these cases, the drive should be for improved quality of services thereby demonstrating better value for money.

An example of the sort of considerations that are relevant to discussions with the clinical director in order to improve the service in obstetrics and gynaecology in the local provider hospital is given in Box 8.8.

Planning for savings

Fundholders are able to use any savings that they make from their fund to improve the services that they provide for patients. Such improvements may include:

- buying additional operations from hospitals
- providing a greater range of services on the practice premises
- purchasing additional equipment
- expanding practice premises
- buying additional activity
- employing extra staff

Any savings made by practices are subject to validation by the Audit Commission and may be carried forward in the GP fundholding accounts for up to 4 years.

Savings can be considered either as:

- planned, where the value of total contracts set is less than funds made available to the practice
- fortuitous, eg where an underperformance trigger is indicated on a cost and volume contract.

Planned savings should have been identified and assessed in the annual health plan, together with a statement of the use to which the savings will be put.

Dealing with under/overexpenditure

Underspending may result from a number of circumstances.

- A fundholder may make savings in particular areas, for example the application of a new prescribing policy.
- There may be unplanned savings, eg if a provider underperformed on a cost and volume contract.
- The original calculation of the fund may have been inaccurate.

If the underspending is due to incorrect setting of the level of the fund, the practice is permitted to keep what is not spent as savings; however, the level of the fund is reviewed in subsequent years.

It is quite possible that an overspending may be on one or more elements of the fund that have been out of the practice's control, and this is not an example of mismanagement. These elements could include:

- an unanticipated, significant increase in list size, affecting both pre-scribing and referrals
- a significant increase in the number of high-cost patients on the practice list; these patients may need high-cost drugs or expensive elective surgery
- errors or discrepancies in either the data or the costs used by the RHA as the basis for setting the level of the fund.

In each case it is important for the practice to have good documentary evidence to support its case for additional funding.

References

1. Pirie A and Kelly-Madden M (1994) *Fundholding: a practice guide, second edition*. Radcliffe Medical Press, Oxford.

9 | Health Planning

Health planning can be considered to be any decision-making process concerned with managing change to ensure the better provision of future services. It means deciding now what to do later. The process consists of:

- analysing the current situation
- formulating objectives
- deciding on strategies and tactics to bring them to fruition.

These steps have all been examined previously in this book and are as true for health planning as they are for strategic business planning.

Doctors are inherently suspicious of any system that challenges their clinical autonomy. In order to develop services within current resource constraints, however, GPs are being encouraged to consider the wider perspective and appreciate that their decisions are fundamental to the proper management of resources. The purpose behind their involvement is to develop a set of common goals and objectives to which the GPs are committed together with fellow DHA/FHSA providers. This requires the fullest information on the cost, quality, quantity and availability of the essential components of various clinical procedures and services.

One of the major obstacles to the integration of GPs into the planning process has been the absence of a common language among planning participants. Clinicians are not trained in resource management and budgetary analysis techniques, while managers often lack the technical skills to appreciate the clinical dimensions of the problem. The presence of GPs brings a relevant casemix dimension to the solution, and their contribution is, therefore, extremely valuable. Once the integration of clinicians into the planning activity is achieved, it is important to encourage them to look at the broader perspective of their activities and to reflect on the manner in which their decisions have wider implications for the provider/population.

A further obstacle to progress has been the nature of the GP's job, which understandably involves a great deal of clinical practice. Any involvement in planning/management is therefore seen as being performed at the expense of patient care/contact. GPs thus require recognition of their involvement. The doctrine of clinical freedom is often used as a defence when one partner departs from the policy/procedure that has been formulated by the practice as a whole. It is important, therefore, that not only one partner but all the partners are able to share the objectives and feel ownership for them.

Fundholding seems to have initiated a gradual change in the general view of GPs with regard to planning, clinical care and resource availability. They are now able to appreciate the greater need for effective and efficient planning in less affluent circumstances. Inevitably, there is a major cultural change involved, as GPs have been trained to consider care and not costs. FHSA managers can have a pivotal role here, as their enthusiasm and commitment may largely determine GPs' attitudes to health resource management. For this to be effective, GPs need to broaden their decision-making horizons, and they need access to accurate, up-to-date information. This raises the issues of the cost of the information technology necessary, and many GPs argue that this money would be better spent on direct patient care.

If GPs are to make a really valuable contribution to the planning activity, however, they need to develop appropriate skills to allow them to operate effectively in this role. These skills would include:

- the concepts of cost–benefit analysis and option appraisal (*see* Chapter 1, page 13)

- computing, budgeting and statistical skills necessary to make properly informed decisions.

Medical audit seems to be an assessment mechanism acceptable to most GPs, as it can be seen to directly improve the quality of patient care and individual outcomes. By promoting discussions between peers, clinical practice is reviewed and standards may be questioned/reappraised. The development of medical audit has allowed clinical care to be reviewed in a systematic manner by consideration of the procedures involved in diagnosis and treatment. This can now be extended to include the consumption of resources compared with outcome and the effects on the quality of life for the patient. The result of this is assurance for FHSA managers and GPs alike that the highest possible standard of care/service provision is being achieved within the total resources available.

Planning can be considered in three basic ways:

- top down planning, in which the FHSA/DHA sets goals and plans for all GPs (fundholders and non-fundholders) to implement, eg childhood immunization programmes

- bottom up planning, in which individual practices determine goals based on what they believe they can achieve and submit these to the FHSA/DHA for approval

- goals down/plans up, in which the FHSA/DHA sets broad districtwide targets in conjunction with GPs, but allows individual practices to develop plans to achieve these objectives.

The last model is much recommended, but can only be achieved by close and harmonious relationships between the practice, the FHSA and the DHA.

Object-oriented analysis and health care planning

When faced with the above scenario health care planning is not a subject with which many clinicians in primary care feel happy. They feel instinctively that they wish to deal with patients and their clinical problems, and that planning should be left to others. This attitude is best described as 'mural dyslexia' – failure to see the writing on the wall. If clinicians wish to see services develop in the way that they feel is appropriate, however, they must take responsibility for the planning of those services. It is often useful to take an 'inside-out' approach, whereby focusing on a specific clinical problem allows principles to be defined which can be applied elsewhere.

Object-oriented analysis[7] and the clinical process model[8], which uses object-oriented methodology, allow a new way of looking at old problems. A 'black box' approach can be adopted, whereby the focus is on the outcome of a process rather than the structure or process itself.

To illustrate this approach, an everyday example can be developed – that of the video recorder. Many families in the UK own and use a video recorder. They understand that one of its purposes is to record television programmes/films onto blank videotapes. It is also understood that in order to record onto a blank tape, the machine will require programming. This task is carried out with more or less success, and many people in this country have learnt the skills required to successfully record the desired programmes. The outcome of the process – to record and watch programmes subsequently – can be achieved without knowing how the machine actually converts television signals into magnetic tape records. This is true of many of the 'black boxes' encountered in everyday life – people have learnt how to use them, but have only the most rudimentary knowledge of their internal workings.

Some examples of how this technique can be applied in health care planning are considered below.

Chronic care

To follow up a patient suffering from a chronic condition, a history has to be taken and an examination, perhaps an investigation, and possibly an operative procedure will have to be completed. These are often repeated at previously decided intervals. For example, a patient with known carcinoma of the bladder might every 3–6 months:

• be asked about symptoms, particularly haematuria

• be examined

• undergo cystoscopy and bladder biopsy

• receive diathermy to any suspicious lesions.

Each of these stages can be thought of as a 'black box'. Each requires different skills to perform and to achieve the desired outcome. Although they may not necessarily be able to understand or perform the process, all clinicians would be able to utilize the information gained – the outcome.

Shared care

If the example of a patient with a torn knee cartilage is considered, application of the 'black box' principle leads to identification of the following stages:

• history and examination

• magnetic resonance imaging

• anaesthetic check

• technical procedure

• rehabilitation.

The current position is that the GP performs history-taking and examination and possibly arranges for magnetic resonance imaging. The hospital performs the rest (often repeating magnetic resonance imaging).
    The desired position is that GPs should:

• perform history-taking and examination

• buy magnetic resonance imaging

- buy anaesthetic check
- buy technical procedure
- manage rehabilitation (this can be broken down into its own constituent parts).

In order to look in depth at the processes of referral and shared care, it is necessary to look at some of the concepts that underpin the clinical process model.

Object of care

This can refer to:

- individual patients
- a population of patients.

This is of immense importance to GPs, who have legally defined responsibilities for their lists of patients. GPs have to provide care to all patients when they are seen, and also organize care so that the defined population is served. Historically, the ethos of general practice was that each GP did his/her best for each individual patient at the time of consultation. GPs today, however, have to balance their responsibility for each patient with their overall responsibility for their defined practice population.

Establishment

- 'An organized body maintained for a purpose'.

An establishment can be anything from a laboratory or clinical team to a nation state. It is important to realize that while clinical standards can be agreed between two clinicians, contracts within the NHS, though not legally binding, have to be agreed between two establishments, eg a fund-holding practice and an NHS trust hospital.

Accountability

- The authority under which an action is performed is represented by an accountability.

An accountability is an agreement that authorizes the carrying out of an action. It is set up between two parties. One party commissions the other;

the second party is accountable to – responsible to – the first for the actions undertaken with the authority of that accountability.

A single accountability can also describe the circumstance of a clinician or an establishment being responsible for the care of a patient over a period of time, eg as defined by a particular illness, however prolonged. That single overall accountability governs the entire period during which the clinician or establishment has a responsibility towards the patient, however slight that responsibility might be and however prolonged the intervals between consultations.

During this period of time, a number of separate consultations, both out-patient and in-patient, can take place. Each consultation is not only governed by the single overall accountability, but can itself involve a number of other accountabilities to cover admissions and/or particular procedures. Each of these accountabilities is confined to the limits of the individual consultation.

When the patient is recorded as having left the clinician's care without a provision for further consultation having been defined, then the single overall accountability ceases.

More than one accountability can govern the performance of an action, for example:

- the patient's formal consent
- the hospital appointment of the clinician
- the contract that will determine payment
- the necessary qualifications and accreditation of the clinician.

These multiple accountabilities are reflected in the relationship between two parties or establishments (patient/GP, GP/consultant, or patient/ consultant) that provides authorization for an action to be carried out.

The areas of particular interest to clinicians are those between a patient and his doctor(s).

- The signing of a form FP1 signifies that a GP has agreed to provide general medical services to that patient. Within the terms of service for patients this means that, subject to certain geographical limits, the GP must arrange for the provision of medical care at all times.

- When a patient attends hospital, there is no formal contract set up between patient and consultant, unless an operative procedure is to be carried out, for which legal consent is obtained.

The grey area that needs clarification arises when a GP asks a consultant for an opinion in regard to a patient's health. Is the accountability that should operate at that time:

- between patient and GP
- between patient and consultant
- between GP and consultant?

Referral

When an accountability is recorded as being proposed, this proposal initiates the process of setting up the accountability that is recorded, eg 'plan: refer to X' is a record of a proposed accountability[8].

- The process of establishing the accountability is initiated by communicating with the party that is to be commissioned, eg by letter.
- The party to whom the patient has been referred can accept or decline – the process is completed or abandoned.
- If abandoned, the action of establishing the accountability can be replaced with a different party to be commissioned.
- Once completed, an accountability is in place; time points of action (start and conclusion) can be recorded.
- When the patient is seen by the consultant, the proposed action becomes an implemented action.

Including accountability as an action allows it to be viewed as a process. The substance of an accountability – what the contract is for – is found in the relationships that are defined as a result of the proposed process. These relationships can relate to:

- the specific actions for which the accountability represents the authority
- the performer
- the time point
- the location.

When the initiation of a referral is completed, a further accountability can be inferred between patient and consultant: once the consultant has accepted the referral he has a duty of care with respect to the details of the referral. This duty usually has little professional or legal responsibility attached to it at first, but these aspects become more substantial as soon as the consultation takes place and the patient is more directly involved.

Examination of this area will show that it is both possible and eminently sensible for an accountability to be set up between GP and consultant before patients become involved and shared care commences.

This is of great value in clarifying the difference between hand-over of care and transfer of care.

Hand-over of care

This is the easier of the two to define. In this situation the GP has no immediate responsibility for the care of the patient, eg, when a general anaesthetic is being administered. In practical terms it also happens whenever a patient is in hospital, eg if a patient suffers a heart attack while in a hospital, treatment will be given without reference to the GP. Such situations are implicitly recognized as being outside the scope of general medical services.

Transfer of care

In this situation only some aspects of the care of a patient are transferred. It is less easy to deal with unless the situation has been fully discussed beforehand. Which areas of care are transferred depends on the clinical scope of the post-holder to whom the patient is being transferred (*see below*).

Post and clinical scope

• The accountability between an establishment and a post governs the clinical scope of the post.

The clinical scope defines the protocols that the postholder will be employed to provide. For each protocol specified, the required period of availability can be stated, as well as the number of times it can be used.

In other words, clinical scope describes the range of responsibilities and services to be provided by each GP. Many complex technical procedures and investigations can only be provided by a consultant. Other activities, eg taking a history, examination, interpretation of test results and confirming that a patient is fit to return to normal duties, can be provided by either a consultant or a GP. Formalizing clinical scope may mean that clinicians do not perform certain tasks, even though they are capable of doing so.

Location

• This is the geographical place where actions or protocols are, have been, or will be carried out.

Consideration of location can have a major impact on the way that services are provided.

- If a complex action is performed at a number of different locations, then one separate location is recorded for each component action that contributes to the parent action.

- If the protocol (or guidelines) that are agreed define the minimal standards to be met, and the competence of those who participate in the management of such patients is acceptable to all parties, then provided the data collected can be shared and made available on a practical time-scale to all parties, the location of such collection is irrelevant.

Protocol

It is generally considered that procedures are performed in accordance with what the clinician understands is possible. This may consist of the clinical knowledge of how to observe or measure a particular characteristic, or how to intervene in an attempt to achieve a particular end.

The performance of any procedure is regarded as being the implementation of one or more distinct protocols. Individual protocols can be defined and distinguished by a number of properties, including:

- circumstance of use

- expected outcome

- necessary resources.

These properties can be referred to when planning and scheduling procedures.

Within the clinical process model, the term 'protocol' has been chosen rather than 'technique' because its popular usage carries a sense of etiquette, an understanding of how things should be done. A narrower usage is sometimes found in clinical care to describe how complex but well-defined procedures should be performed.

Protocol as a term, however, has a legal connotation. Use of the term guidelines (of how to observe and manage) may be more acceptable to clinicians wishing to take the first steps towards the formal sharing of care.

Skill

In addition to having accountability, it may be necessary for a performer to hold the skills that are required for the implementation of a protocol.

The ability to perform a protocol is seen as distinct from the authority to perform it.

Skill also relates to knowledge of the specificity and sensitivity of any particular procedure or protocol, particularly of laboratory tests. Those who perform such tests must be aware of these issues. Those who are sent the results, whether in general practice or hospital medicine, need to use them – the outcome of the 'black box' procedure – and may accept the results in a clearcut yes/no fashion (as is the current practice).

Planning

Plan process rules

Planning offers the opportunity for recording actions (as proposed actions) in advance of their being performed, and for organizing all the actions planned for a patient, including those proposed by different parties. All component proposed actions required as a result of planning can be listed in terms of the plan structure associated with each one. The sequence in which proposed actions are to be implemented is determined by plan process rules.

A number of people or teams can be involved in making plans for a patient. Attempted integration of these plans may reveal conflicts and/or duplications. Further planning, repeated often if necessary, can lead to the creation of new rules which resolve the conflicts and/or duplications.

Result of planning

The substance of a clinical plan is made up of proposed actions which can take the form of:

• procedures
• proposed accountabilities
• proposals for further planning sessions.

When planning a proposed action, the protocol required may already be covered by an existing clinical scope. An accountability therefore already exists to provide authority for the implementation of the action, and a new one is not required.

Shared care – the current situation

Existing accountabilities

Accountabilities are already in existence before a patient registers with a GP. The ones discussed here are those that are set up with the secondary services (Figure 9.1 and Box 9.1). These accountabilities may have been set up by the contracts that the DHA has with the provider unit or the fundholding practice.

These accountabilities are therefore between establishments and apply to objects of care in the population sense.

Other existing accountabilities include those between:

- hospital trust and consultant, as outlined in the consultant's contract (which defines clinical scope)

- FHSA and GP in the terms of service of that GP

- the practice, ie all the partners, and each individual GP as defined in the practice agreement or partnership law.

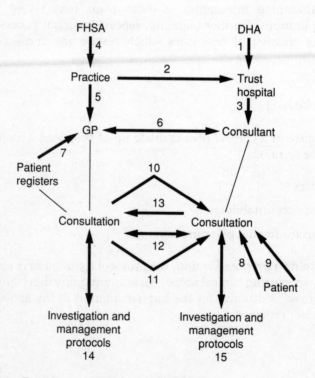

Figure 9.1   Existing accountabilities in shared care.

Box 9.1   Shared care – current accountabilities

		Set up
1 DHA–trust	Contract (purchaser/provider)	Annually
2 GP fundholder–trust	Contract (purchaser/provider)	Annually
3 Trust–consultant	Contract of employment	Tenure or fixed term
4 FHSA–practice	Terms of service with each GP	Once – modifiable
5 Practice–GP	Partnership agreement	Once – modifiable
6 GP–consultant	Clinical standards, implicit, subject to audit, non-enforceable	
7 Patient–GP	Registration	Once
8 Patient–consultant	Admission via accident and emergency department	New or ongoing
9 Patient–consultant	Self-admission	Ongoing
10 Patient–consultant	Emergency admission	Ongoing
11 Patient–consultant	Referral to out-patient department	Once or repeated
12 Patient–consultant	Ongoing care in out-patient department	Once or repeated
13 Patient–GP	Discharge	Once or repeated
14 Patient–GP	Investigation and management	Once or repeated
15 Patient–consultant	Investigation and management	Once or repeated

Emergency admission

This is an implemented action that can take place in the following ways, without the patient being registered with any GP.

- The patient attends an accident and emergency department and is admitted from there.
- The patient admits him/herself directly to hospital.

In the first instance, the accountability that is set up between the patient and the consultant may be a new one or it may be the continuation of an existing accountability. If the patient has permission for direct admission to the ward, this constitutes the continuation of an existing accountability.

Patient registration with GP

This is the setting up of an accountability between an object of care and the GP. The accountability has a starting point.

Observation protocol

Emergency admission via the GP is an implemented action, which arises either implicitly or explicitly from an observation protocol. Thus:

- implicitly: 'I don't like the look of you; you should go to hospital'
- explicitly: 'Your peak expiratory flow rate is less than 120 litres/minute, and your pulse is above 100 beats/minute – you require admission'.

The point to be made here is that many of the behaviours that take place do relate to a protocol, but not to one that the GP could readily verbalize.

Once a patient has been admitted to hospital the GP has no immediate responsibility for the care of that patient. This will remain true for as long as the patient continues as an in-patient. This represents hand-over of care.

Referral

The GP does not have immediate responsibility once the patient is seen in the hospital out-patient department. Some referral letters will state precisely what the GP requires from the accountability that is to be set up; others leave the matter entirely in the hands of the consultant – 'please see and advise'. It should be remembered that referral is a planned action, which means that the GP is in a position to request the accountability that is set up.

Transfer of care

In practice this does not fully take place at the present time. Transfer of care exists in the sense that consultants restrict themselves more to their clinical scope and tend to treat the patient less. For example, a physician may still diagnose depression, but will inform the GP of the situation and leave management, including the decision on whether to make a referral to a psychiatrist, to the primary care physician. Within their own clinical fields, however, consultants work to their own standards.

Discharge

This is of two types:

- to follow up, ie the accountability with the consultant remains in force
- to the GP, with the accountability between patient and consultant ending.

Location and shared care

The fact that the care of the patient takes place in separate locations, which are only linked on a routine basis by letter for communication of management of the patient, leads to the fact that at present independent protocols of both observation and intervention take place.

Shared care – a view of the future

The way forward for shared care appears to be the adoption of protocols that take into account the clinical scope of each post-holder (doctor). In other words, accountabilities 10–15 from Box 9.1 would merge into an all-embracing investigation and management protocol (Figure 9.2 and Box 9.2). This means that the patient would be cared for under the same protocol whether this were undertaken in primary care or in the secondary sector (Box 7.8, accountability 10).

This in turn would allow the separate accountabilities 10–15 outlined in Figure 7.1 to be planned and coordinated. If the two establishments could be linked electronically, data entered at either location could be used in achieving the standards laid down in a protocol common to both sites.

If it were also accepted that clinicians at *either* site were competent to undertake the subsidiary protocols that made up the overall protocol, then location would become truly irrelevant. Shared care would then be represented by a three-way accountability: GP–patient–consultant.

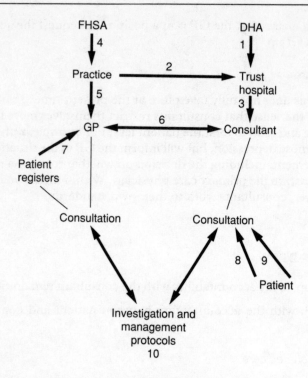

Figure 9.2 Possible future accountabilities in shared care.

The health plan

Many reasons can be given for a modern general practice becoming involved in planning, and a similar range against it. These are summarized in Box 9.3.

The health plan itself:

- shows how the organization intends to move from the present to proposed positions
- identifies the preferred option
- informs those who are interested
- is evidence of activity and a caring philosophy
- can be used to obtain resources
- offers marketing and public relations opportunities
- is a source of information
- is a tactical weapon for change.

Box 9.2   Shared care – possible future accountabilities

			Set up
1	DHA–trust	Contract (purchaser/provider)	Annually
2	GP fundholder–trust	Contract (purchaser/provider)	Annually
3	Trust–consultant	Contract of employment	Tenure or fixed term
4	FHSA–practice	Terms of service with each GP	Once – modifiable
5	Practice–GP	Partnership agreement	Once – modifiable
6	GP–consultant	Clinical standards, implicit, subject to audit, non-enforceable	
7	Patient–GP	Registration	Once
8	Patient–consultant	Admission via accident and emergency department	New or ongoing
9	Patient–consultant	Self-admission	Ongoing
10	GP–patient–consultant	Shared protocols	Ongoing

The detailed contents of a health plan should include:

- a set of commissioning and financial objectives for the next financial year

- the reasons why these objectives can and should be met, in view of the needs assessment of the practice population

- the management activities necessary to meet these objectives

- a detailed plan of action (implementation plan) to put the programme into effect

- contingency plans in the event that the commissioning assumptions or the practice resources change during the implementation period

---

Box 9.3   Advantages and disadvantages of participating in health planning

Advantages	Disadvantages

Advantages

- Provides structura framework for developments
- Better coordination of effort
- Identifies and quantifies all available resources
- Diminishes crisis management
- States policies
- Provides information
- Neutralizes bias
- Involves GPs in a formal system
- Explains decision criteria
- Permits judgement of outcomes
- Evidence of innovation
- Develops performance standards
- Demonstrates intent and commitment
- Permits effective allocation of resources
- Specifies monitoring/evaluating criteria and mechanisms

Disadvantages

- Time-consuming
- Induces complacency
- Consumes resources in its preparation
- Creates unsatisfiable expectations
- Soon becomes out-of-date
- Time lag from preparation to approval of plan
- System not easily accessed by GPs due to technical jargon
- Crystallizes partisan interests

- provisions for evaluation of the commissioning performance both during and by the end of the financial year.

Health planning for general practice is still in its infancy and will undoubtedly develop as experience is gained in both the preparation and the implementation of plans. This development will clearly be easier if practices work closely with their DHA and FHSA purchasing/planning colleagues.

References

1. Stott NCH, Davis RH (1979) The exceptional potential in each primary care consultation. *Journal of the Royal College of General Practitioners* **29:** 201–5.

2. Grol R (1993) Development of guidelines for general practice care. *British Journal of General Practice* **43:** 146–51.

3. *The health of the nation* (1991) HMSO, London.

4. NHS Directorate (1992) *Caring for the future – the pathfinder.* The Welsh Office, Cardiff.

5. Partridge M (1994) Asthma: guided self management. *BMJ* **308:** 547–8.

6. Drummond N *et al.* (1994) Integrated care for asthma: a clinical, social, and economic evaluation. *BMJ* **308:** 559–63.

7. Martin J, Odell J (1992) *Object-oriented analysis and design.* Prentice Hall, London.

8. NHS (1992) *The clinical view of the common basic specification. The Cosmos project clinical process model version 2.0.* NHS Management Executive, Birmingham.

10 | A Structure for Business and Health Plans

Even though each general practice is unique and plans are written for specific purposes, a standard format with essential elements is expected. This ensures that all the significant matters are addressed in turn, yet still allows the creation of a document that is particular to the practice. Business plans, health plans, fundholding plans and development plans are terms often erroneously used interchangeably. While their purposes may differ, however, the process and contents are often similar.

It is recommended that any plan is kept as free from jargon as possible, as terms with which they are not familiar will confuse the audience at which the plan is directed. Not every practice will be able to complete a full business plan unaided. The attempt will be a valuable learning experience, however, which may also save expenditure on accountancy fees. This guide is intended to be free from much of the jargon associated with strategic planning in the commercial environment.

It is important that the principal aim for the production of each individual plan is both clearly stated and understood. In this way, the unique characteristics of each practice will be captured in the document, and the objectives will be more meaningful. It is worth remembering what type of audience the ultimate readers will be. The audience can be a disparate group:

- owners – the partners themselves
- investors – bank or building society
- stakeholders – the FHSA, people with whom the practice trades, employees.

Each practice is a stakeholder in many other businesses, including the FHSA. Large companies, eg J Sainsbury or Marks and Spencer, will not trade with others unless they have considered their business plan. The bank manager will be more interested in practice financial arrangements than in an activity analysis, whereas the FHSA will have a clinical/service interest.

The plan writer must bear the reader in mind at all times. This is where some distinguishing features between 'health' and 'business' planning appear.

General outline of the plan

Although each plan will be unique, it is helpful if a similar format is adopted, which makes it easy for the plan to be followed. The sections normally included, in their order of appearance, are shown in Box 9.1. It is useful to examine each of these sections in a little more detail.

Index

It is not so important how the plan is indexed as long as the index has a logical structure that enables the reader to see at a glance what the plan contains and where individual items of information are located. This allows for ready cross-referencing and avoids the need to duplicate information unnecessarily. The index is the guide that takes the reader logically through the plan.

Box 10.1   Components of business/health plans

- The index, which is the guide to what follows

- A summary or overview of the plan, to attract the reader to finish the document

- The purpose of the plan, which makes clear the reasons for preparing the plan

- The history and details of the practice, showing that it is capable of managing change

- Development proposals, which quantify the purpose in terms of time and resources

- Summarized financial information, confirming that the fuller implications have been thought through

- Supporting appendices, leaving the above sections free of detailed information

---

Summary/review

This is meant to be an abstract of the document. It will necessarily be concise, but it must be written in a way that is sufficiently attractive to make the reader want to read the whole of the document. These first two sections cannot be written until the rest of the document has been completed.

Statement of purpose

This is where the principal aim of the plan is developed and formulated. Everything else provides supporting information to secure that aim. Clearly, there will be a difference of emphasis depending on whether the intention is, for example, to secure funding for a new computer system (a practice business plan) or convince the local hospital to provide additional resources for a service used by the practice (the fundholding/health plan). After giving the reader a concise statement of purpose, further examination of the details is undertaken with the overall goals clearly in mind.

If an application is being made for resources from the reader, it is important to:

- quantify these

- state the use to which they will be put

- make an assessment of the benefits that will accrue to all parties from this course of action.

Clearly, financial outcomes are more easily measured than health gain, but the imperfections in the outcome measures need not detract from making sensible predictions.

The plan needs to demonstrate that the partners, or perhaps the extended primary health care team, have the abilities successfully to manage the practice as a business/fundholder. The reader will be looking to find the appropriate mix of professional skill and expertise, practice track record and management environment that will be necessary to succeed.

Practice details

This section is the opportunity to provide more details of the practice. In particular, the history of the practice and the financial arrangements underpinning it should be outlined. The intention is to provide the reader with sufficient information to understand how and why the practice has reached its present position. This section should therefore not be expansive, but sufficient to convey the key points.

It is important, however, for the writer to make clear what type the practice is, in terms of the range of services offered, to a sufficient level of detail that enables the reader to distinguish why this practice is successful but others are not. There could, for example, be a unique method of service delivery or an advantageous use of technology specific to the practice.

Clearly, it is important to emphasize the areas where the practice is pre-eminent or superior to others, but care must be taken to avoid confusing a reader who has no particular medical knowledge. It may be helpful to include the practice leaflet as one of the appendices.

Development proposals

To this point, the document has detailed the practice history, current position, and the overall goal. This section involves projecting present and proposed services into the future. It is therefore much more difficult to write, and the underlying assumptions will be subject to careful scrutiny. Proposed developments should be shown to be appropriate, realistic and credible. This section must be as objective as possible.

In the wider business world, this section would include marketing considerations. Even in terms of general practice, it is possible to contemplate a market for health care, though this may be limited to comparison with the immediate competitors of the practice. This issue was considered further in Chapter 6.

Patient satisfaction surveys are becoming more common, and the writer may know a great deal about why patients use the practice in preference to another, enabling a statement of competitive advantage to be made. This section should also identify how the practice intends to capitalize on the advantage.

Marketing factors outline the potential growth for the business, and this is particularly true of the post-1990 contract world. Patients need to be attracted to the increasing services that are provided for them – services of all shapes and sizes. It is important to demonstrate how additional or unique services are incorporated into the plans for expansion of the business.

Summarized financial information

This section may be limited to an analysis of the practice accounts or the calculation and disbursement of the fund, but it should only include information that is relevant to the development proposals. Simply photocopying the accounts may not be adequate, as it is important that the accounts are interpreted for the reader in order to convey the correct message. The accounts show historical data and are the basis on which to build the project into the future. Clearly, in the preparation of a health plan, the GP fundholding accounts would be used.

The summary allows the preparation of cash flow forecasts on monthly, quarterly and annual bases and the development of projected income and expenditure accounts for these periods, together with balance sheets for the relevant year ends.

This may be the area where support is required from a financial advisor or specialist health planner. If the practice has a computer that allows spreadsheet models to be created, it is possible to make a start, which can be later refined. The advantage of spreadsheet models is that a number of scenarios based on various input factors can be developed without laborious workings by hand. In addition, this section should include a key commentary on the interpretation of the spreadsheets.

Comparisons may be made between the practice this year and the previous two years, and against the national and local averages. Typically, this would include capitation and item of service income, mean profit per full equity partner for practice purposes, or work-load, deprivation and activity data for health planning purposes.

Essentially, this section should summarize the forecasts and key assumptions. Detailed projections should be included as an appendix. It should be remembered that this is a projection into the future, and need not be calculated to the last penny, instead rounding off the figures to thousands or, at least, hundreds of pounds.

Supporting appendices

This section should include all the relevant details that supports the assumptions, analysis and predictions included in the previous sections. It will inevitably be different for each practice, and the writer must judge what is appropriate to include. This section should not be used to 'pad out' the plan, so only information that is directly relevant to the other sections of the plan should be included.

Writing the plan

Although it may seem rather simplistic to state, it is best to start with a blank piece of paper and think through the issues involved. If the FHSA or others have a proforma document to follow, then this is helpful. Historical data need to be readily to hand to supply the details that allow an evaluation of where the practice is now and how it arrived there. It should be remembered that in producing a plan for the future, the practice needs to demonstrate that it is capable of achieving the proposed goals. Goals can be expressed in terms of:

- financing a project
- dealing with issues of computerization
- introducing a practice-based service as a consequence of fundholding.

Goals need to be:

- objective
- measurable
- realistic.

Having identified where the practice is and where the partners want it to be, it is possible to set benchmarks against which achievement/success can be measured. In doing so, an estimate is required of the resources needed to achieve the plan, be they financial, staff, accommodation, or skills.

The reader of the plan will undoubtedly challenge the underlying assumptions. The plan will be more likely to succeed if the writer considers some of the questions that the reader may raise.

- Are the plans achievable/worthwhile?
- What are the long-term effects of failing to implement the plans?
- Do the financial forecasts support the proposals?
- Are the assumptions conservative/optimistic?
- Have alternative options to the proposal been considered?

Considering these in advance may save the practice substantial effort later on and helps the writer to produce an effective narrative. The narrative is equally as important as the figures or schedules, and they need to be consistent with one another. This allows the practice the opportunity to state its case and justify the use of the underlying assumptions.

The plan is about the management of the partners' business (or the fund), so it is important that all the partners contribute to and convey their enthusiasm and commitment to the reader. Depending on the purpose of the plan, it may be appropriate to involve others in its creation, eg the practice manager or fundholding staff. While many can contribute to writing the plan, the setting of practice goals should remain the responsibility of the partners.

Box 10.2   Necessary steps in the production of business/health plans

- Deciding who is going to coordinate and write the plan

- Determining what information needs to be collected within the practice and from external advisors

- Deciding how to collate the information for each topic/section and when to start jotting down ideas

- Ensuring that the information is in a logical format and a skeleton index is prepared

- Commencing writing and remembering to be concise

- Rereading and rewriting the plan until a satisfactory version is prepared

---

Only one person can effectively collate the data and write the whole plan. Individual sections could be separately written, provided that a coordinator remains in overall editorial control of activity. The plan is not meant to be a voluminous document and should be as brief as possible, consistent with its purpose. It should be remembered that the reader may be busy, so fine detail needs to be consigned to appendices, leaving the main plan to be a comprehensive statement. The necessary steps in the production of the plan are given in Box 10.2.

Having reached the final version, it is important to challenge the assumptions for reasonableness and to ask someone else to review it. This could be a partner who was not heavily involved in the preparation, the practice accountant, or another trusted colleague. Whoever it is, it is important that the plan is read from the viewpoint of the ultimate reader. This is the last opportunity to make improvements to the contents and presentation of the plan, so it should be used wisely.

Items specific to health plans

The structure recommended above is generic for business-type plans. The annual health plan requires more specific components, the data from which are aggregated by the FHSA. The health plan is geared more to reviewing:

- the practice and the population it serves

- the range of services currently provided

- a limited number of practice objectives.

The text has to be supported by:

- a detailed breakdown of purchasing intentions
- proposals for the management of the prescribing element of the fund
- action plans for each of the key initiatives.

A typical health plan is given in Appendix H.

Proforma SWOT analysis

Internal

Strengths	Weaknesses
Opportunities	Threats

External

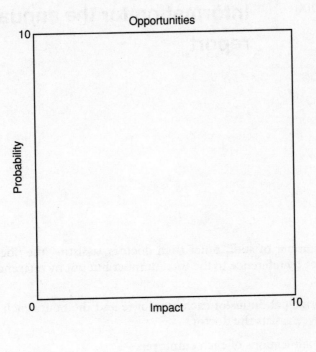

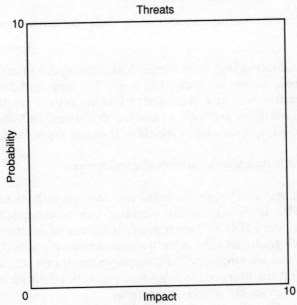

Information for the annual report

Staff

- The number of staff, other than doctors, assisting the doctor in his practice by reference to the total number but not by reference to their names.
- The principal duties of each employee and the hours each week the employee assists the doctor.
- The qualifications of each employee.
- The relevant training undertaken by each employee during the preceding 5 years.

The total number of staff assisting the doctor can be calculated by looking at the payroll, as can the hours they work. The principal duties of each employee will have to be ascertained by looking at their job descriptions. If job descriptions are not available, the audit will already have highlighted a major deficiency which will require urgent action.

- Do all your staff have contracts of employment?

Employees may not yet be qualified nor have undergone any relevant training. This is an area where planning can be extremely valuable. Enquiries to the FHSA will elicit what qualifications are deemed necessary for each grade, and also what training courses are available for each of the staff that are employed. The employment of new staff will require evidence that the prospective employee's qualifications are suitable for employment as set out in job descriptions.

An audit of the number of courses that staff have been sent on during the last year may be required in order to show that employees have reasonable opportunities to undertake training with a view to maintaining their competence.

The future reimbursement of receptionists may depend on them having been trained and having subsequent inservice training. If the practice is being reimbursed for its receptionists in the future, it may have to adhere to these minimal standards. In-service training may, however, be viewed as a means of valuing and motivating the practice staff.

- What staff training do you have planned in the next year?

Premises

The following information is required about the practice premises:

- any variations in relation to floor space, design, or quality since the last annual report
- any such variations anticipated in the course of the forthcoming period of 12 months.

Answering this section with another entry of 'not applicable' may be the stimulus for undertaking a new cost-rent scheme

- What premise developments are planned?

Referrals

The following information about the referral of patients to other services under the NHS Act 1977 during the period of the report is required:

- referrals by the GPs to specialists
  —the total number of patients referred as in-patients
  —the total number of patients referred as out-patients
  by reference in each case to whichever of the following clinical special-ties applies and specifying in each case the name of the hospital concerned:
  —general surgical
  —general medical
  —orthopaedic
  —rheumatology (physical medicine)
  —ear, nose and throat
  —gynaecology
  —obstetrics

—paediatrics
—ophthalmology
—psychiatry
—geriatrics
—dermatology
—neurology
—genitourinary
—radiology
—pathology
—others (including plastic surgery, accident and emergency,
  endocrinology).

• the total number of cases of which the doctor is aware (by reference
  to the categories listed above) in which a patient referred himself to
  services under the NHS Act 1977.

If information has to be presented in a certain way, it is much easier to
do so if has been recorded in that format in advance. This again answers
the 'where are we' question, and comparison with other practices defines
the limits of 'who do we want to be'. If the practice referral pattern is
outside the normal range, some action on referral practices may be
considered. The practice must determine who admits patients, whether
it is all done by partners, by trainees, by other principals in a local
cooperative, or by deputizing services, and it must determine how the
admissions are recorded.

A central bed bureau, if present, will record information, but if
admissions are direct the doctor concerned will certainly have to make a
separate record. The most foolproof methodology is to create an admission book, which is retained in the practice and which is kept up-to-date
with the appropriate information. Similarly, those practices that maintain
a full computer record will be able to audit the appropriate Read Codes
for emergency and elective admissions. The same principles apply to
out-patient attendances, though these are far more likely to be generated
solely within the practice.

If admissions from the practice are centralized through a secretariat,
these staff are in an ideal position to keep the appropriate records. If the
practice GPs generate referral letters, either by hand or through a
computer system, the onus is on them to make sure that their individual
records are kept up-to-date.

Estimation of self-referral by patients to hospital is extremely difficult.
The only obvious method of recording is to audit discharge letters and
to compare discharges against admissions, looking for patients who were
not admitted by the practice and disaggregating those who enter the
system via an accident and emergency department.

• What are the practice referral rates in these various categories?

External commitments

A report is required of the GPs' other commitments as medical practitioners with reference to:

- any posts held
- all work undertaken, including in each instance the annual hourly commitment.

These requirements can be met as a minimum by the GPs providing clearly descriptive information. All of this information, however, has an impact on the practice, and it may act as a focus or trigger for the practice to reconsider this aspect of clinical commitments.

- Do the outside commitments of the practice represent value for money?

Consumerism

This comprises the nature of any arrangements whereby the GPs or their staff receive patients' comments on the provision of general medical services.

- Does the practice have such arrangements?

Should it if it does not? Examples of a suggestion and complaints leaflet and a patient's charter are included in Appendix D and Appendix E, respectively.

Prescribing

The following information is required in respect of orders for drugs and appliances:

- whether the practice has its own formulary
- whether the GPs use separate formularies
- the practice's arrangement for the issue of repeat prescriptions to patients.
- What steps has the practice taken towards a formulary?

Information technology considerations

The following constitutes a checklist of questions for consideration before the introduction of information technology into the practice.

Organizational considerations

- How will the new technology actually change the nature of the practice business?
- What use will be made of the new information available?
- How will this affect the flow of information?
- What will be the impact on the number and type of jobs?
- How will the organizational structures be affected?
- How will the overall physical arrangement of the space need changing?
- Is there full partnership commitment?
- Is there full employee commitment?
- Will the organization climate accept change?
- Who will take the initiative for piloting the change?

Job considerations

- Which jobs will be affected?
- Are jobs likely to disappear?
- What new jobs will be created?

- What functions will be merged?
- How many, and which, jobs will be changed?
- Can new or remaining jobs be enriched or enlarged?
- Are there problems of boredom?
- Do the jobs create any kind of stress?
- How can the adverse factors be eliminated?

Job design

- Can new jobs be designed so that the tasks combine together to make up satisfying jobs?
- Is each job organized so that tasks are not too tiring or repetitive?
- What feedback is provided on performance levels?
- Do jobs contain sufficient variety?
- Do jobs contain an element of challenge?
- Do employees have responsibility for their own work?
- Does the job ensure that the skills of job-holders are well used?

Participation considerations

- Are people involved in issues that affect them?
- Is everyone being consulted specifically about the introduction of new technology?
- Are their views properly represented?
- Is involvement early enough?
- Is involvement regular enough?
- What account is taken of what people say?
- Can the system be altered to accommodate suggestions for improvement?

Communication considerations

- What are the existing means of communication and consultation?
- Can problems be identified early enough?
- Do people have a chance to express their views?
- Are they told what is expected of them?
- Are they told how well they are doing?
- Do they have a chance to talk to colleagues?
- Are there regular communications meetings?

Technical considerations

- What objectives does the equipment need to meet?
- What are the volumes of work?
- What are the time-critical pressures?
- What equipment is available to meet the defined operational needs?
- What equipment should be considered?
- How reliable is the equipment?
- Are servicing arrangements satisfactory?
- Can the equipment be up-graded to meet the future needs of the practice?
- How does the equipment fit in with other systems within the practice?
- What are the cost implications?
- Can the practice afford it?
- What will the practice save?
- Are the costs worth the gain?
- Should the practice buy, rent, or lease?
- How flexible is the system to future changes in need?
- What is the lifespan of the equipment?

Ergonomic and safety considerations

* Is the new equipment safe?
* Does it provide proper levels of comfort?
* Is it tiring to use?
* Is lighting adequate?
* Are there problems of screen reflections or glare?
* Is there sufficient room for all operations and maintenance to be carried out safely?
* Are seating arrangements satisfactory?
* Is ventilation good enough?
* Are noise levels acceptable?
* Is there any fire risk?
* Are any electric safeguards, eg isolation switches, required?
* Are 'clean' power lines required?

Recruitment and training

* How will the change affect recruitment, selection, and retirement patterns?
* What kind of people will be needed for the future?
* What extra skills will be required?
* What training will be needed to meet these skill requirements?
* How can existing people be best used, by training or redeployment?
* Who will need retraining?
* What type of training is available, and from whom?
* How can increased responsibility be given to people?
* Are some people not suited to the new system, either physically or temperamentally, despite all efforts to retrain them or redeploy them? What should be done about them?

Evaluation

- Does the system meet the objectives set for it?
- Is it efficient?
- Is it cost-effective?
- Will it meet the practice's future needs?
- What modifications/upgrading are necessary?
- Has the quality of working life been improved?
- What further changes of personnel are called for?
- What lessons can the practice learn from the changes?

Model suggestions and complaints scheme

Comments, suggestions or concerns about services provided by Ely Bridge Surgery: A patient's guide

Our approach to good service

While we aim to provide a high-quality service at all times, we recognize that there may be occasions when our services fall short of what you may expect from us.

This leaflet has been prepared to explain the practice's procedure for dealing with any suggestions or concerns from patients regarding the services received. Any comments made by patients are regarded by us as valuable aids in sustaining and improving the quality of service that you receive.

We hope that nothing occurs while you or your family are in our care that makes you concerned. Should you feel that you have reason to be unhappy, however, we will deal with it in a proper manner.

At the time you are attending the surgery or receiving services at home, please feel free to discuss any fears you may have with the doctor or member of staff who is dealing with you. It is best to express concern at this stage so that you can be reassured or further action can be taken.

We are pleased to receive comments about health authority or social services staff attached to our practice, but because we are not responsible for these services, it will be necessary for us to forward your comments to the appropriate body.

Complimentary comments on good services

Should there be any aspects of our service that you feel are particularly good we would like to know, and in this event you may write to the practice manager. We will use this opportunity to bring your satisfaction to the attention of the individual concerned.

If you have a problem with our services

- Please discuss your concerns while you are receiving treatment, or as soon as possible thereafter. We can then improve the situation.

- If you do not want to discuss it with the doctor or member of staff treating you, ask to speak to the practice manager. Details of your concern will be noted, and we will arrange for you to discuss the matter with another doctor at a mutually convenient time.

- Alternatively, you may write directly to the practice manager. Please keep copies of any letters you send us. We shall deal with your letter promptly and send you an acknowledgement within 7 days.

- In the first instance your concern will be reviewed by the doctor you usually see, who may wish to discuss the matter with you further. If so, we shall make an appointment for you at a mutually convenient time.

- If you are still unhappy after this discussion, the matter will be referred to the most senior partner who has not been involved in the discussion so far, for further consideration.

If you remain dissatisfied with our response

If you are unhappy with the reply you receive, you should discuss the reasons for this with the Family Health Services Authority. Remember you are free to change to another doctor's practice if you wish without reference to us. The Family Health Services Authority can advise you of other doctors in the area.

The general manager of the Family Health Services Authority will arrange for a member of the authority's staff to consider your problem further. The National Health Service has a very detailed procedure for making formal complaints about your doctor, and the Family Health Services Authority will be able to advise you further. You should contact the General Manager, South Glamorgan Family Health Services Authority.

Patient's charter – an example

The patient's charter for Ely Bridge Surgery

- We are committed to giving you the best possible service. We cannot achieve this aim without the support and involvement of you, the patient.
- We need to work with you in partnership to build on the high standards we have already achieved.
- Please help us to help you.

Your rights and responsibilities when using practice services

- You will be treated as an equal in the care and attention you receive.
- You will be treated as an individual and will be given courtesy and respect at all times, irrespective of your ethnic origin, religious belief, personal attributes, or the nature of your health problems.
- Following discussion you will receive the most appropriate care given by suitably qualified people. No care or treatment will be given without your informed consent.
- Within the limitations of the law, patients are entitled to see their medical records. This should be discussed first with the doctor, and a fee may be chargeable for this service.
- We will give you full information about the services we offer. Every effort will be made to ensure that you receive the information that directly affects your health and the care being offered.

- People involved in your care will give you their names on request and ensure that you know how to contact them. You should let us know if you change your name or address.

- It is our job to give you treatment and advice. In the interest of your health it is important for you to understand all the information given to you. Please ask us questions if you are unsure of anything.

- We need help too. Please ask for a night visit only when you feel it is truly necessary. Home visits by the doctor are only for patients who are too ill to visit the surgery.

- Please do everything you can to keep appointments, and tell us as soon as possible if you cannot. Remember, your cancelled appointment can be given to someone else. Be ready to tell us of your past illnesses, medication, hospital admissions and any other relevant details.

- We will provide you with information about how to make suggestions or complaints about the care we offer. We want to improve services and will therefore welcome any comments you have. Please ask for our separate leaflet. You may discuss your comments with the doctor whom you normally see, or if it is not relating to your health, with our practice manager.

Our principal quality standards for general medical services

- As a minimum, our practice accommodation will be maintained to the standard necessary by National Health Service regulations, health and safety requirements and the recommendations of the Family Health Services Authority.

- Appropriate facilities for disabled patients will be provided, including access to and within the building, including toilet areas.

- No patient who is waiting to be seen should normally have to stand to wait.

- Where patients are being seen via our appointments system, they will normally be seen within 15 minutes of the appointment time or be given an appropriate explanation for the delay. This standard does not apply to our Cathedral Road branch surgery, where no appointment system operates, or to patients who are being seen at short notice for urgent reasons outside our normal appointments system. Remember, Saturday surgery is for emergency cases only.

- Requests for repeat prescriptions are not accepted by telephone for reasons of safety and confidentiality. Requests for repeat prescriptions are accepted at any time, and any requests received by 12.00 noon will be available for collection after 4.00 pm on the same day. Requests received after 12.00 noon will not be available for collection until after 4.00 pm on the next normal working day.

- Patients seeking advice between 6.00 pm and 8.30 am will receive a clinically appropriate response from the doctor on call. Remember that this is an emergency service for conditions that are too serious to wait until the next working day. Always leave a telephone number with the doctor's answering service.

- Information is freely available to patients on the current range of services available. Please enquire at reception.

- Whenever possible, incoming telephone calls will be answered within 1 minute. At the busiest times (between 8.30 and 9.15 am) all lines may be engaged and patients are requested to leave non-urgent calls until later in the day.

- The practice operates as a primary health care team and patients are encouraged to contact the practice nurse or health visitor directly without reference to the doctor, when this is appropriate. The team meets at least quarterly to discuss the range of services provided to practice patients.

How you can help yourself and us

You can play your part in helping Ely Bridge Surgery to give you a better quality of care by:

- being informed about your health or condition, and by asking questions and discussing your care with the doctor or nurse. This will help you to make decisions based on better knowledge and understanding

- knowing your medical history and whether you are allergic to any medicines

- answering questions about your health frankly and honestly

- being considerate towards other people using the surgery and towards staff running our services

- taking care of any loaned equipment and returning it promptly when no longer required

- accepting our advice on vaccination, immunization and health screening programmes

- managing your own health and well-being by maintaining a healthy lifestyle, eg taking regular exercise and eating a varied, healthy diet

- ensuring that requests for home visits are made before 10.30 am and are only made when you are too ill or medically unfit to attend an appointment at the surgery.

Other information

The information we provide to patients includes:

- the *Patients' Guide to Ely Bridge Surgery* (our practice booklet)

- booklets and leaflets on different aspects of health care lifestyles (either displayed in the surgery or by request to the practice nurse or health visitor)

- an abridged annual report, published in July, which details our performance in the commissioning of health services with relation to patients' charter standards

- copies of the patients' charter for the NHS in Wales (either displayed in the surgery or by request to the receptionist)

- a statement of our principal quality standards for general medical services which is displayed in the surgery

- guidance on how to express your views on the services provided (separate leaflet available from the reception desk)

- details of how to obtain access to your medical records (separate leaflet available from the reception desk). Please note that a fee may be charged for this service.

We need your help if we are to continue to improve our services to you. We would welcome any comments or views about your experiences.

Sample job descriptions and person specifications

Job description

Job title: Fund manager
Responsible to: Partnership
Liaises with: Regional Health Authority, District Health Authority, Family Health Services Authority, provider units (including directly managed units, NHS trusts and private hospitals) and other GP fundholding practices

Summary of main responsibilities and activities

The fund manager will be responsible to the partnership for the overall management and development of the fund within the context of practice activities.

He/she will be responsible for implementing the management, structural and other changes necessary for the future successful operation of the whole range of fund activities.

Operating context

The Government White Paper *Working for Patients* introduced the concept of fundholding for GPs and the post has been created to meet the challenges of fundholding within this practice. The relationship between the partners and the fund manager will be crucial and is perceived to be akin to that with a non-clinical partner.

It will remain the responsibility of the partners to plan, individually and collectively, the global clinical activity that provides the identified level of health care necessary for the practice's patients.

The role of the fund manager will be to predict, calculate, interpret and explain the financial implications of the planned changes. The effect of this will be to incorporate business planning into the global delivery of care, such that the partners have access to all necessary information on financial outcomes before making changes in their clinical activity.

The best interests of individual patients remain paramount at all times.

Specific responsibilities

General management

- Responsible for the successful and efficient implementation of fund management within the practice organization. This will include establishing appropriate and necessary monitoring arrangements and reviewing the management controls.

- Responsible for managing all the fund activities and providing effective leadership and direction.

- Responsible for effective liaison with RHAs, the FHSA, provider units, other GP fundholding practices, the medical profession (BMA, LMC etc) and other interested parties.

- Corporate responsibility as business advisor to the partners for the overall policy and organization of the fund activities.

Planning

- Prepares strategies and short-term plans which reflect clinical and non-clinical aims, in collaboration with partners, in respect of training, fund management and service development.

Staff management

- Responsible for the management of all staff appointed to practice posts, in support of fundholding.

- Ensures that effective personnel policies and practices exist, including staff and management development, to maximize the effective use of resources within the scope of the fund.

Financial and fund management

Responsible for providing and maintaining an effective financial system and managing resources including:

- routine operation of the fund involving accounting, double-entry book-keeping, invoicing and payment systems, both manual and computerized

- integrating the elements of the fund with practice clinical policy (based on sound understanding of the mechanisms by which the fund has been derived and the reasons and logic that underpin clinical decision-making) and arranging virement between elements as required

- delegation of appropriate tasks to employed staff, and training/educating staff to achieve these

- incorporating the activities of attached staff that impact on the fund, to achieve desired outcomes by clarification/understanding of their role

- undertaking such detailed negotiations with the FHSA as the partners may delegate in respect of the staff and drugs elements of the fund

- preparation and reconciliation of fund accounts for partnership approval, prior to payment

- undertaking such detailed negotiations with the DHA as the partners may delegate in respect of the diagnostic/referrals and community services elements of the fund

- establishing, with the partners, the terms of the service agreements with provider units and devising mechanisms for effective monitoring and review of same; examination of alternative sources of supply

- examining invoices for accuracy and initial investigation of discrepancies

- acting as the principal point of contact with the RHA, the DHA and the FHSA on all matters pertaining to the fund

- preparing such regular and ad hoc reports as may be necessary for the effective management and audit of fund activity

- ensuring such effective liaison with practice financial advisors (banking, accountants etc) as is required to oversee and audit both the fund and the practice accounts (where relevant to GPFH).

Monitoring and review

- Monitors the standards and operation of services provided for the practice by employed and attached staff, including professional staff and takes necessary action.

- Takes an active role in the overall evaluation of fund management in conjunction with RHA-appointed consultants.

- Prepares for and participates in an accountability review process undertaken by the partnership in conjunction with the FHSA and the RHA.

- Ensures that all procedures are as defined in the relevant RHA/DoH fund management guidelines.

Quality

- To be responsible for the implementation of all quality issues pertaining to fundholding.

Person specification

Position: Fundholding manager

This is intended to enable the right person for the job to be found in the fairest possible way.

Personal attributes

- Minimum – to be available at unorthodox hours and work effectively under a range of pressures. Possession of a high standard of general intelligence, ability to communicate orally and in writing and have good numerical ability.

- Desirable – creates strong impression; top 10% for general intelligence, considerable ability to communicate orally and in writing with numerical ability in top 5%.

Education

The successful candidate is preferred to have a relevant degree, eg in management, accounting, or business management, or professional qualifications, together with evidence of continued education since graduation.

Experience, training and skills

- Minimum – proven managerial experience in a multiprofessional organization; ability to plan, organize, coordinate and control and work under pressure. At least 5 years' health service experience, preferably in primary health care.

- Desirable – particular knowledge and skills in the areas of general management and financial management. Good communications; interpersonal and diplomatic skills. Working knowledge of computerized systems in general practice.

Personality

- Minimum – motivated to achieve and to manage others effectively; ability to adjust; ability to innovate and manage change; sense of vision towards strategic goals.

- Desirable – mature and stable personality; strong leadership and staff management skills; ability to communicate at all levels and to be persuasive in argument with excellent influencing skills.

Age

- Desirable – none specified, subject to attainment of experience, training and skills, as mentioned above. It is unlikely, however, that a candidate younger than 30 years of age will have met the above requirements.

Job description

Job title: Information officer
Responsible to: Business/fundholding manager
Liaises with: Partners, hospital information and medical records departments, hospital and FHSA finance departments, computer system suppliers/maintainers

Summary of main responsibilities and activities

To establish and maintain the patient database, such that fundholding processes may be undertaken, validated and summarized, to conduct audits of the database and to maintain database integrity.

Principal responsibilities

Fundholding services

- To create, amend and maintain the clinical system database in respect of all hospital referral activities, to include:
  - set up of providers' details on computer system
  - creation of service agreements
  - referral protocols/practices
  - pricing data.

- To reconcile activity reported by practice and by provider, such that any discrepancies are resolved to the satisfaction of the practice.

- Daily operation as system administrator of both the referral ledger and nominal ledger, to include backing up the system, closing monthly or other period accounts and producing reports as required.

- To ensure that all patient activity is recognized by the system, including completion of data entry by clinicians and administrative staff.

- Routine operation of the fund involving accounting, double-entry bookkeeping, invoicing and payment systems, both manual and computerized.

- Delegation of appropriate tasks to employed staff and training/educating staff to achieve these.

- Examining invoices for accuracy and initial investigation of discrepancies.

- Preparing such regular and ad hoc reports as may be necessary for the effective management and audit of fund activity.

Information services

- To monitor the financial performance of the staff element of fundholding, by reference to payroll costs and authorized budget, to prepare reconciliation and investigate discrepancies.

- To monitor financial and prescribing performance of the practice in relation to the authorized budget for the drugs and appliances element of fundholding.

- To conduct such other audits of activity recorded on the database as may be requested or delegated.

- To ensure that system data is recorded/reported in as efficient a manner as possible.

Computer system management

- To ensure that the performance of the system is optimal and that users are aware of amendments/updates/developments as necessary.

- To maintain relevant error, fault and repair logs and to act as principal point of contact with computer suppliers.

- To ensure the security of the system, including password access to various levels of the system, taking and storage of tape backups of system data and the physical security/integrity of the system.

Secondary responsibilities

- To fulfil any other duties appropriate to the grade as the partners or fundholding manager may from time to time delegate.

Addendum

The practice is presently undergoing a period of change and the job description must be seen in this context. The above duties are therefore neither prescriptive nor comprehensive and may be subject to change as developments occur.

The implications of such changes will be discussed with the incumbent to ensure that objectives remain reasonable and achievable. The post will be subject to a participatory system of evaluation, such that attainment of joint objectives is regularly reviewed/assessed, at least on an annual basis.

Some interview questions

- Modesty and space must have prevented you giving a full picture in your curriculum vitae. Please outline the things you had to leave out that you feel might be relevant to our needs.

- Have you developed any special techniques for managing people?

- How do you plan your criticism of subordinates? Please give an example.

- What have you been criticized for in the last year? Do you think it was valid?

- What irritates you in the work-place?

- What makes you less effective?

- When you leave your present job, what will your boss say?

- What changes in your present environment would stop you applying for other jobs?

- What are your two key strengths and weaknesses?

APPENDIX

Model GP fundholder
health plan

Contents

Section 1: Introduction

This health plan outlines the purchasing intentions of Ely Bridge Surgery GP fundholders for the financial year 1994/95. These plans are based on the firm foundations established with providers of health care in the first 3 years of fundholding and seek to extend the quality of care provided to patients by the practice. Although GP fundholding is a relatively new concept, the practice firmly supports the principles outlined in the strategic intent and direction for the NHS in Wales, and our plans remain patient-centred with a clear drive to deliver health gain.

To this end, the practice has decided to continue to introduce incremental changes in the manner in which some services are delivered. It has been possible to do this as GP fundholding encourages innovation and resource flexibility within the overall framework of patient care. Since the practice commenced fundholding we have been able to collate data of greater depth and accuracy on morbidity and patient needs. This information has been incorporated into our planning activity and the following proposals reflect this.

It should be noted that, at the time of writing, the practice has no firm budget for hospital services expenditure in 1993/94. It has been accepted by the FHSA and the Welsh Office that there have been significant flaws in both the original data collection exercise and the first 2 years' activity data, particularly relating to completeness of information. It has not been possible to remedy these inadequacies to date, but these are expected to be resolved during 1993/94.

We recognize that the entire thrust of GP fundholding is to improve services to patients, and we continue to work closely with our consultant colleagues in the hospitals to build relationships and to ensure that GP fundholding remains patient-centred and clinically directed. Fundholding to date has been principally about establishing and building relationships between the practice and providers. During 1994/95 we intend to examine more carefully the quality of service provided for our patients. Our underlying philosophy remains that patients will continue to receive the care they need irrespective of the current administrative problems associated with GP fundholding.

Partners: Geoffrey Morgan
Peter Edwards
Huw Charles
Karen Santos
Trevor Thompson
Helen Lindsey
Jane Evans

Service Development Manager: Stephen Jones

October 1993

Section 2: Health plan summary

GP fundholding covers only part of the overall delivery of health care services to practice patients and relates to the following discrete areas in 1994/95:

- referrals to consultant out-patient services
- certain elective procedures in a discrete number of specialties, provided on both in-patient and day case bases

- defined direct access services, eg physiotherapy
- diagnostic tests and investigations, eg radiology
- domiciliary consultant visits
- community nursing services.

It is our intention that these activities in combination with the general medical and other services provided by the practice, will ensure that all patient contacts that are directed by the practice are:

- Health gain focused – we seek to add years to life through reduction of risk factors contributing to premature death, and life to years by promoting individual awareness and encouraging improvement in well-being
- Patient-centred – we shall continue to value our patients as individuals and manage our services to provide the optimum care that each individual requires to the highest standard achievable
- Resource-effective – as far as we are able and as is compatible with our practice objectives and clinical responsibilities, we shall deploy our resources in a cost-effective manner.

The following sections of the health plan relate only to the six discrete areas mentioned above. In order that there should be no significant adverse change affecting provider units, the practice intends to continue to contract with the existing providers in the main. The changes proposed remain marginal in cost terms, but offer significant health gains for patients and provide measurable alternative delivery mechanisms where the benefits may not accrue in the same financial year.

Since April 1993, provider hospitals have been able to provide the practice with data on the practice waiting list. During the course of 1993/94 we have discussed the list with provider units and expressed our concern on the delay in receiving of suitably detailed data. A full analysis of our patients on out-patient and in-patient waiting lists was performed at the end of March 1993, analysed by provider. This information is being used to monitor the achievement of the patients' charter guarantees. It is to be regretted that information technology systems at provider units do not permit a comprehensive validation to take place on other than a quarterly basis.

The practice still has limited information on the number and times of patients on various waiting lists, and this is insufficient to construct an overall picture. With regard to in-patients and day case patients, some provider units are failing to distinguish between chargeable and non-chargeable procedures, and both DHA and practice waiting lists are therefore subject to an undetermined margin of error.

Section 3: Practice and population summary

The practice has seven partners operating from a main surgery in Ely and a branch surgery in Cathedral Road, Cardiff. The practice population of approximately 12 500 patients is predominantly social class IV and V, while the area served is a largely disadvantaged council estate. The age–sex profile is shown in Annex A. It remains the aim of the practice to continue to review the benefits and costs for general practice fund-holding status for both the patients and the GPs.

The following objectives underpin the practice purchasing strategy for 1994/95:

- to remain at the forefront of general medical practice and maintain our position as one of the leading practices in South Glamorgan
- to provide a full and comprehensive preventive, curative and palliative health care service for our patients
- to maintain and improve the quality of our existing health care services
- to support innovative and appropriate methods of delivering health care services to our patients
- to play an important part in the development of local strategies for health and measurement of health gain in the coming years
- to balance the objectives of providing optimum health care services with that of achieving improved cost control
- to enhance management, communication and organizational skills to lead to a more efficient and effective practice
- to continue to deliver job satisfaction to everyone associated with the practice in terms of time, commitment, individual performance, professional reputation and financial reward
- to extend and develop our relationships with secondary care clinicians, other GP fundholders, the FHSA, the DHA, provider units, NHS trusts and the Welsh Office.

Section 4: Current service provision

The practice received an initial allocation of £1 742 000 in 1993/94 (not including amendments due to changes in costing methodology) and this is constituted from:

Hospital services expenditure	£706 000
Community nursing services expenditure	194 000
Prescribing costs	716 000
Staff costs	126 000
	£1 742 000

It is expected that the hospital services element will purchase, based on 1992/93, the following levels of activity for practice patients:

- 222 in-patient procedures

- 142 day case procedures

- 1144 out-patient referrals

- 6645 diagnostic tests and investigations

- 235 direct access services

- 4 domiciliary consultations.

The principal method of contracting will be cost and volume, with 5% trigger values based on 1992/93 activity, and the pattern of referrals will remain broadly consistent with our historical basis. The majority of our referrals are to the University Hospital of Wales, while Cardiff Royal Group and Llandough Hospital NHS Trust constitute the balance. Consistent with one of our key initiatives, the practice intends to make Llandough Hospital NHS Trust our first choice for general surgical referrals. Other referrals will continue to be sent to appropriate locations within South Glamorgan.

Waiting list management remains a problem due to the delay of information received from our principal provider. This is due to both the delay between activity taking place and being reported, and the long response time in provider validation of practice-generated activity queries. For the first 3 months alone, some 500 queries remain unresolved. The waiting list projections for 31 March 1994 (shown in Annex D, tables 1, 2 and 3) must therefore be viewed in the light of this. The practice does not believe that sufficient activity and pricing information is available to cost the projected waiting list.

Section 5: Key practice initiatives

The following three key services will be developed, based on the experience gained in financial year 1993/94, in discussion with clinical colleagues.

Prescribing

The practice recognizes that repeat prescribing constitutes a significant proportion of its overall drug costs, and it is intended to examine a find, stop and commence policy in order to tackle the problem. This approach will examine respiratory drugs in the first instance, and certain drugs will be targeted. All patients who receive medication with a specific Read Code will, over time, have that drug altered to another clinically equivalent drug with a different Read Code. Were the practice able to persuade our computer suppliers to modify the software to permit a drug-specific find and replace for the practice population, it would be considerably easier to undertake this exercise, which will currently have to be undertaken on a patient-by-patient basis and will be extremely time-consuming.

Surgery at Llandough Hospital NHS Trust

This is an area that offers considerable scope for improvement of the clinical service to our patients. It is anticipated that waiting times could be reduced with a concomitant increase in numbers treated. It is vital, however, that the overall quality of service does not suffer. Patients require a comprehensive service, and it is intended, therefore, to continue discussions with the provider unit to purchase a comprehensive package of care. Joint guidelines of care are being established with a consultant surgeon, and discrete procedures within the specialty will be reviewed prior to a major shift to this mode of treatment. This will ensure an effective patient-centred service that is broadly resource-neutral.

Cardiovascular disease

The establishment of a reduce/stop smoking clinic in the surgery during 1994/95 will enable patients to reduce/stop smoking and develop alternative strategies to cope with stress. Protocols are currently being developed for our SOPHIE health promotion programme, and success will be compared with our prescribing initiatives (Annex B).

Section 6: Purchasing intentions for 1993/94

For reasons explained previously, this section and the appended tables are significantly less informative than we would wish. We have provided all the information that is available to us, indicating trends and intentions where exact figures are not available.

Volume of activity

Activity levels remain consistent with the fund allocated to the practice and represent the continuance of our historical referral pattern.

Historical and future provision of services

Services have been provided by the University Hospital of Wales, the Cardiff Royal Group of Hospitals, the Llandough Hospital NHS Trust, Whitchurch Hospital and its community mental health team and St Lawrence's Hospital, Chepstow. Fewer than a dozen referrals are made elsewhere, these being mainly to London teaching hospitals. As a consequence of the information deficiencies in the first 3 years, the practice is unable to make any significant alteration to its referral pattern in 1994/95. The same providers will be used, as outlined above, except where services may be transferred between providers as a result of revised management arrangements in South Glamorgan. As before, the majority of our activity will be undertaken within the District.

The practice will not significantly change its pattern of referrals compared with previous years. The level of service (yet to be agreed) for 1993/94 and that planned for 1994/95 will be firmly based on the actual activity in 1992/93 and not on the extrapolation of the simple data by which the fund was originally calculated. In 1992/93 the value of the hospital services element was scaled up to reflect the under-recording of activity during the data collection exercise. It has not yet been possible to finally complete this exercise, due to the change in the costing methodology used by provider hospitals. It was expected that there would be a clear move away from block contracts to cost and volume contracts during 1993/94, but this has not been possible due to the protracted negotiations with the providers over costing methodologies. It remains our intention to develop this approach as more meaningful information becomes available during 1994/95.

As during this year, cost per case contracts will be made with providers elsewhere in the UK where in the GP's clinical opinion this is to the advantage of the patient. The number of such referrals in 1994/95 will not be significant and is in line with our plans to develop responsive local services in conjunction with consultant colleagues.

Practice age–sex profile

All	Male	Female	Male		Female
1	0	1		100+	
7	0	7		95–99	
38	9	29		90–94	*
86	17	69		85–89	***
210	74	136	***	80–84	*****
237	96	141	****	75–79	******
481	205	276	*******	70–74	***********
473	212	261	*********	65–69	**********
487	238	249	*********	60–64	*********
587	289	298	***********	55–59	***********
607	309	298	************	50–54	***********
766	385	381	***************	45–49	****************
730	401	329	****************	40–44	**************
903	471	432	******************	35–39	*****************
1147	586	561	***********************	30–34	**********************
1276	636	640	*************************	25–29	*************************
1031	444	587	*****************	20–24	***********************
729	373	356	***************	15–19	**************
893	443	450	*****************	10–14	******************
1012	527	485	*********************	5–9	*********************
1109	580	529	***********************	0–4	***********************
12810	6295	6515		TOTALS	

Prescribing of medicines and appliances

The practice continues to prescribe as clinically indicated, taking due regard of the cost and effectiveness of the drugs utilized. It is intended that a baseline will be established for those patients who are diagnosed as suffering from asthma. Those patients who are being treated with β-agonists alone and those patients who are using inhaled or oral steroids in their therapeutic regimen will be expressed as a numerical ratio and compared with national norms to look at the relative performance of the practice.

Anxiolytics and hypnotics

The total amount of these drugs will be compared with the prescribing of antidepressant drugs and will be expressed as a ratio. This will provide a baseline that will be more sensitive to the needs for the practice population than merely recording the total number of prescriptions issued.

Antibiotics

The practice prescribing of antibiotics will be linked to our initiative on pathology reporting. We have discussed with colleagues in pathology the introduction of more specific feedback on organisms, and it is intended to make our prescribing more specific and sensitive in this respect.

Non-steroidal anti-inflammatory drugs

It is the intention of the practice to identify which groups of patients are taking these drugs and to examine possible alternatives.

Ulcer-healing drugs

The practice will seek to identify those patients who may benefit from triple therapy, which will allow cessation of treatment in the longer term.

Health promotion

The major thrust of cardiovascular health promotion within the practice is an anti-smoking strategy. As well as setting up anti-smoking clinics it is intended to:

* audit the baseline of Nicotinell prescribing
* monitor lipid screening and, in conjunction with the pathologist, monitor the number of abnormal results that have been discovered.

Asthma and diabetes

Care programmes will be enhanced by the use of SOPHIE, which is our computer health promotion guideline programme, for the correct collection and utilization of data about patients with these conditions.

Timetable for development of practice formulary

The *Grey List* (*see* Health Plan 1993/94) is already in place. This consists of the first choice for prescribing in each of the therapeutic groups for those drugs that contribute high cost and/or high volume in each category. This is recommended for partners, but remains mandatory for trainee GPs and locum practitioners.

Our approach to generic prescribing has its roots in the Grey List (*see* above) and we intend to regularly compare generic prescribing with the FHSA average.

Monthly meetings are already in place with each partner responsible for a specific therapeutic area, to review the prescribing activity of the practice and also any new developments in that area. In these monthly meetings the practice's own prescribing information is utilized as well as that from PACT.

As the practice wishes service to remain patient-centred, great care will be taken in the consideration of our 'find and replace' policy (*see* Section 5: Key practice initiatives). Any replacement drug will be acceptable to patients in term of quality, quantity and appearance of the drug, and patients will be given information that the change is taking place.

It is expected that each of these initiatives will reduce our prescribing costs, but this is difficult to quantify at this time.

Key initiatives: action plan

Prescribing

Aim

- to reduce costs associated with repeat prescribing

Responsibility

- Dr T Thompson
- Mr S Jones

Target outcomes/products

- To develop an acceptable find and replace methodology
- To apply this methodology to inhaled drugs for respiratory disease

Timetable

- To commence by April 1994

Audit and review

- To compare drugs prescribed in this therapeutic group on a regular basis in comparison to 1993/94 quarter 4 prescribing

Surgery at Llandough Hospital

Aim

- To develop joint guidelines on clinical care

Responsibility

- Dr PH Edwards
- Mr DA Aubrey

Target outcomes/products:

- Written guidelines for joint management of patients with general surgical problems

Timetable

- June 1994

Audit and review
Not applicable

Cardiovascular disease

Aim

- To provide an enhanced service to patients who wish to stop smoking

Responsibility

- Dr H Lindsey
- Practice nurses
- District nurses

Target outcomes/products

- Appropriate clinic to be established
- 50% of patients attending will still have stopped smoking 3 months afterwards

Timetable

* To be established by April 1994

Audit and review

* Ongoing measurements of smoking status of attendees

Procedures financed from the fund

Table 1: In-patient procedures

Table 2: Day-case procedures

Table 3: Out-patient procedures

Table 1 In-patient procedures.

Procedure	Waiting at 31 March end year 94	Total volume	Volume to be obtained from each provider unit				
			UHW	CRG	LLAN	WHIT	Other
Category: 01 Ophthalmology Total	20	20	20				
001 Squint							
002 Chalazion							
003 Pterygium							
004 Ectropion, entropion, and ptosis	2	2	2				
005 Glaucoma							
006 Obstruction of nasolacrimal duct							
007 Extraction of cataract	14	14	14				
008 Corneal graft	4	4	4				
009 Laser treat for vascular retinopathies							
Category: 02 E.N.T. Total	42	42	42				
010 Myringotomy	1	1	1				
011 Insertion of grommet							
012 Mastoidectomies							
013 Stapedectomy							
014 Tympanoplasty	8	8	8				
015 Labyrinthectomy							
016 Septoplasty	2	2	2				
017 Sub-mucous resection of septum							
018 Polypectomy	2	2	2				
019 Ethmoidectomies							
020 Turbinectomy	4	4	4				

Table 1 continued

Procedure	Waiting at 31 March end year 94	Total volume	Volume to be obtained from each provider unit				
			UHW	CRG	LLAN	WHIT	Other
021 Cautery of lesion of nasal mucosa	1	1	1				
022 Puncture of maxillary antrum	4	4	4				
023 Drainage of maxillary sinus	2	2	2				
024 Exploration of frontal sinus							
025 Tonsillectomy	21	21	21				
026 Adenoidectomy	4	4	4				
027 Pharyngoscopy							
028 Laryngoscopy							
029 Laryngectomy							
030 Block dissection	4	4	4				
Category: 03 Thoracic surgery Total							
031 Bronchoscopy (with or without biopsy)							
032 Biopsy/excision lesions lung/bronchus							
033 Lobectomy/pneumonectomy							
Category: 04 Cardiovascular surgery Total	4	4	4				
035 Valv or isc dis of heart (ex. neon & inf)	4	4	4				
Category: 05 General surgery Total	83	83	60	2	21		
036 Partial thyroidectomy							
037 Total thyroidectomy							
038 Thyroidectomy of aberrent thy gland							

Table 1 *continued*

Procedure		Waiting at 31 March end year 94	Total volume	Volume to be obtained from each provider unit				
				UHW	CRG	LLAN	WHIT	Other
039	Salivary gland and ducts							
040	Parathyroid glands							
041	Oesophagoscopy							
042	Dilation of oesophagus							
043	Varices of the oesophagus							
045	Gastrectomy (partial or total)							
046	Vagotomy							
047	Endoscopy							
048	Laparoscopy	4	4	4				
049	Excision lesion of small intestine	2	2	2				
050	Partial colectomy	8	8	4		4		
051	Total colectomy							
052	Sigmoidoscopy	12	12	4		8		
053	Colonoscopy	4	4	4				
054	Exteriorization of bowel							
055	Repair of prolapsed rectum							
056	Anal fissure and fistula	2	2	2				
057	Excision of rectum	16	16	16				
059	Pilonidal sinus	4	4	4				
060	Dilation of anal sphincter							
061	Haemorrhoidectomy	1	1			1		
062	Gallbladder	6	6	4	2			
063	Bile ducts	4	4	4				
064	Mastectomy							

Table 1   continued

Procedure	Waiting at 31 March end year 94	Total volume	Volume to be obtained from each provider unit				
			UHW	CRG	LLAN	WHIT	Other
065 Excision/biopsy of breast lesion	1	1	1				
066 Repair of inguinal hernia	9	9	5	4			
067 Repair of femoral hernia							
068 Repair of incisional hernia	2	2	2				
069 Varicose veins stripping/ligation	8	8	4	4			
070 Surg treatment of ingrowing toenail							
071 Excision/biopsy of skin or subc tiss							
072 Lymph node excision biopsy							
Category: 06 Urology Total							
073 Cystoscopy	30	30	5	25			
074 Dilation of urethra/urethrotomy	20	20	4	16			
075 Urethroplasty							
076 Open repair							
077 Prostatectomy (open or tur)	1	1		1			
078 Hydrocele							
079 Orchidopexy							
080 Male sterilization							
081 Circumcision	1	1	1				
082 Varicocele							
083 Removal of ureteric/renal calculus							
084 Lithotripsy							
085 Nephrectomy	8	8		8			

Table 1 continued

| Procedure | Waiting at 31 March end year 94 | Total volume | Volume to be obtained from each provider unit | | | | |
			UHW	CRG	LLAN	WHIT	Other
Category: 07 Gynaecology Total	67	67	27		40		
086 Oophorectomy/salpingoophorectomy	4	4	4				
087 Ovarian cystectomy							
088 Wedge resection of ovary							
089 Female sterilization	12	12	4		8		
090 Patency tests of fallopian tubes	8	8			8		
091 Hysterectomy (abdominal/vaginal)	12	12	4		8		
092 Myomectomy							
093 D & C	8	8	4		4		
094 Cone Biopsy	12	12	4		8		
095 Colposcopy							
096 Anterior or posterior repair	6	6	2		4		
097 Vulvectomy/partial vulv/vulval biopsy							
098 Marsupialization of barth cyst/abscess							
114 Diagnostic laparoscopy	3	3	3				
115 Eua							
116 Hysteroscopy/endometrial resection	2	2	2				
Category: 08 Trauma & Orthopaedic Total	24	24		24			
099 Intervertebral discs	1	1		1			
100 Therapeutic lumbar epidural inject	1	1		1			
101 Arthroplasty/rev arthrop of hip/knee	10	10		10			
102 Removal of implanted subs from bone	1	1		1			

Table 1 continued

Procedure	Waiting at 31 March end year 94	Total volume	Volume to be obtained from each provider unit				
			UHW	CRG	LLAN	WHIT	Other
103 Upper tibial osteotomy							
104 Arthroscopy	4	4		4			
105 Intra-articular inject/aspiration							
106 Meniscectomy	1	1		1			
107 Osteotomy for hallus valgus/rigidus							
108 Dupuytren's contracture							
109 Carpal tunnel decrompression	2	2		2			
110 Release of trigger finger							
111 Excision of ganglion							
112 Correction of hammer toe	4	4		4			
113 Aspiration/excision of bursa							
Total, all categories	270	270	158	51	61		

Table 2 Day case procedures.

Procedure	Waiting at 31 March end year 94	Total volume	Volume to be obtained from each provider unit				
			UHW	CRG	LLAN	WHIT	Other
Category: 01 Ophthalmology Total	10	18	18				
001 Squint	5	5	5				
002 Chalazion	1	1	1				
003 Pterygium							
004 Ectropion, entropion, and ptosis							
005 Glaucoma							
006 Obstruction of nasolacrimal duct							
007 Extraction of cataract	4	12	12				
008 Corneal graft							
009 Laser treat for vascular retinopathies							
Category: 02 E.N.T. Total	9	45	45				
010 Myringotomy	1	1	1				
011 Insertion of grommet	4	40	40				
012 Mastoidectomies							
013 Stapedectomy							
014 Tympanoplasty							
015 Labyrinthectomy							
016 Septoplasty							
017 Sub-mucous resection of septum	4	4	4				
018 Polypectomy							
019 Ethmoidectomies							
020 Turbinectomy							

Table 2 *continued*

Procedure	Waiting at 31 March end year 94	Total volume	Volume to be obtained from each provider unit				
			UHW	CRG	LLAN	WHIT	Other
021 Cautery of lesion of nasal mucosa							
022 Puncture of maxillary antrum							
023 Drainage of maxillary sinus							
024 Exploration of frontal sinus							
025 Tonsillectomy							
026 Adenoidectomy							
027 Pharyngoscopy							
028 Laryngoscopy							
029 Laryngectomy							
030 Block dissection							
Category: 03 Thoracic surgery Total		8			8		
031 Bronchoscopy (with or without biopsy)		8			8		
032 Biopsy/excision lesions lung/bronchus							
033 Lobectomy/pneumonectomy							
Category: 04 Cardiovascular surgery Total							
035 Valv or isc dis of heart (ex. neon & inf)							
Category: 05 General surgery Total	6	77	36	8	33		
036 Partial thyroidectomy							
037 Total thyroidectomy							
038 Thyroidectomy of aberrent thy gland							

Table 2 continued

Procedure	Waiting at 31 March end year 94	Total volume	Volume to be obtained from each provider unit				
			UHW	CRG	LLAN	WHIT	Other
039 Salivary gland and ducts							
040 Parathyroid glands							
041 Oesophagoscopy							
042 Dilation of oesophagus							
043 Varices of the oesophagus							
045 Gastrectomy (partial or total)							
046 Vagotomy							
047 Endoscopy		41	16	8	17		
048 Laparoscopy							
049 Excision lesion of small intestine							
050 Partial colectomy							
051 Total colectomy		8	4		4		
052 Sigmoidoscopy		5	5				
053 Colonoscopy	1						
054 Exteriorization of bowel							
055 Repair of prolapsed rectum							
056 Anal fissure and fistula							
057 Excision of rectum							
059 Pilonidal sinus							
060 Dilation of anal sphincter	1	1	1				
061 Haemorrhoidectomy	1	1	1				
062 Gallbladder							
063 Bile ducts							
064 Mastectomy							

Table 2 continued

Procedure	Waiting at 31 March end year 94	Total volume	Volume to be obtained from each provider unit UHW	CRG	LLAN	WHIT	Other
065 Excision/biopsy of breast lesion	1	4	4				
066 Repair of inguinal hernia	1	4			4		
067 Repair of femoral hernia							
068 Repair of incisional hernia							
069 Varicose veins stripping/ligation							
070 Surg treatment of ingrowing toenail							
071 Excision/biopsy of skin or subc tiss	1	13	5		8		
072 Lymph node excision biopsy							
Category: 06 Urology Total	4	44	19		25		
073 Cystoscopy		24	4		20		
074 Dilation of urethra/urethrotomy		1	1				
075 Urethroplasty							
076 Open repair							
077 Prostatectomy (open or tur)							
078 Hydrocele							
079 Orchidopexy		1	1				
080 Male sterilization		2	2				
081 Circumcision	4	16	11		5		
082 Varicocele							
083 Removal of ureteric/renal calculus							
084 Lithotripsy							
085 Nephrectomy							

Table 2 *continued*

Procedure	Waiting at 31 March end year 94	Total volume	Volume to be obtained from each provider unit				
			UHW	CRG	LLAN	WHIT	Other
Category: 07 Gynaecology Total	11	58	18		40		
086 Oophorectomy/salpingoophorectomy							
087 Ovarian cystectomy							
088 Wedge resection of ovary							
089 Female sterilization	3	11			11		
090 Patency tests of fallopian tubes							
091 Hysterectomy (abdominal/vaginal)							
092 Myomectomy							
093 D & C		6	6				
094 Cone Biopsy	8						
095 Colposcopy		40	12		28		
096 Anterior or posterior repair							
097 Vulvectomy/partial vulv/vulval biopsy							
098 Marsupialization of barth cyst/abscess							
114 Diagnostic laparoscopy							
115 Eua		1					
116 Hysteroscopy/endometrial resection					1		
Category: 08 Trauma & Orthopaedic Total		7	4	3			
099 Intervertebral discs		4	4				
100 Therapeutic lumbar epidural inject							
101 Arthroplasty/rev arthrop of hip/knee							
102 Removal of implanted subs from bone							

Table 2 *continued*

Procedure	Waiting at 31 March end year 94	Total volume	Volume to be obtained from each provider unit				
			UHW	CRG	LLAN	WHIT	Other
103 Upper tibial osteotomy							
104 Arthroscopy	2	2		2			
105 Intra-articular inject/aspiration							
106 Meniscectomy							
107 Osteotomy for hallus valgus/rigidus							
108 Dupuytren's contracture							
109 Carpal tunnel decrompression	1	1		1			
110 Release of trigger finger							
111 Excision of ganglion							
112 Correction of hammer toe							
113 Aspiration/excision of bursa							
Total, all categories	40	257	140	11	106		

Table 3 Out-patient services.

Specialty		GPFH category code	GPFH treatment type code	Waiting at 31 March end year 94	New out-patient attendances	Total out-patient attendances	Volume of total attendances to be obtained from each provider unit				
							UHW	CRG	LLAN	WHIT	Other
1000	General Surgery	09	2100	190	164	500	182		318		
1010	Urology	09	2101	93	105	164	16	132			16
1100	Trauma & Orthopaedic	09	2110	105	145	236	236				
1200	E.N.T.	09	2120	121	160	416	416				
1300	Ophthalmology	09	2130	51	72	348	348				
1400	Oral Surgery	09	2140	2	4	12	12				
1500	Neurosurgery	09	2150	8	18	48	48				
1601	Plastic Surgery	09	2160	36	42	150	110				40
1700	Cardiothoracic Surgery	09	2170	8	14	28	20		8		
1710	Paediatric Surgery	09	2171	27	36	52	52				
1900	Anaesthetics	09	2190	5	12	30	30				
3000	General Medicine	09	2300	38	68	482	374	14	94		
3010	Gastroenterology	09	2301	13	17	41	41				
3020	Endocrinology	09	2302		4	18	18				
3030	Haematology (clinical)	09	2303	8	18	172	143	29			
3040	Clinical Physiology	09	2304								
3050	Clinical Pharmacology	09	2305								
3100	Audiological Medicine	09	2310								
3110	Clinical Genetics	09	2311								
3130	Clinical Immunology & allergy	09	2313								
3140	Rehabilitation	09	2314								
3150	Palliative Medicine	09	2315								
3200	Cardiology	09	2320	34	52	320	290		30		

Table 3 *continued*

Specialty		GPFH category code	GPFH treatment type code	Waiting at 31 March end year 94	New out-patient attendances	Total out-patient attendances	Volume of total attendances to be obtained from each provider unit				
							UHW	CRG	LLAN	WHIT	Other
3300	Dermatology	09	2330	80	160	325	286		39		
3400	Thoracic Medicine	09	2340	7	56	164			164		
3500	Infectious Diseases	09	2350								
3600	Genitourinary Medicine	09	2360								
3610	Nephrology	09	2361		4	32	32				
3700	Medical Oncology	09	2370								
3710	Nuclear Medicine	09	2371								
4000	Neurology	09	2400	46	54	128	128				
4010	Clinical Neurophysiology	09	2401								
4100	Rheumatology	09	2410	5	24	68	60	8			
4200	Paediatrics	09	2420	39	61	256	137	78	41		
4210	Paediatric Neurology	09	2421		4	14	14				
4300	Geriatric Medicine	09	2430	18	28	104	93	9	2		
5020	Gynaecology	09	2502	95	124	464	278		186		
7000	Mental handicap	09	2700								
7100	Mental Illness	09	2710	85	124	382	96			286	
7110	Child & Adolescent Psychiatry	09	2711								
7130	Psychotherapy	09	2713								
7150	Old Age Psychiatry	09	2715								
8000	Radiotherapy	09	2800								
8100	Radiology	09	2810								
9010	Occupational Medicine	09	2901								
9900	Joint Consultant Clinic	09	2990								
9999	TOTAL	09	2001	1114	1570	4954	3460	270	882	286	56

Table 3 *continued*

Specialty	GPFH category code	GPFH treatment type code	Waiting at 31 March end year 94	New out-patient attendances	Total out-patient attendances	Volume of total attendances to be obtained from each provider unit				
						UHW	CRG	LLAN	WHIT	Other
Diagnostic Tests	10	3001	25	6645	6645	108	792	5745		
Domicillary Consultations	11	4001								
Direct Access Services	12	5001	36	98	235					235

Model health and safety policy

Ely Bridge Surgery attaches the greatest importance to the safety of its employees, patients and visitors. It is the policy of the practice to consider this as a management responsibility equal to that of any other function. Any reference in this document to employees being male should be seen as a means of illustration only. The policy will apply equally to all male and female employees.

In the operation and maintenance of all buildings, equipment, facilities, practices and procedures, it is the duty of the practice to take all reasonably practicable measures to prevent personal injury or risk to health.

Employees have a statutory duty under the Health and Safety at Work Act to take reasonable care of their own health and safety and that of other persons who may be affected by their actions, and to co-operate with their employer in respect of any duty or requirement imposed by law.

In particular it is the personal responsibility of each employee to conform to procedures, rules and codes of practice, and to use properly and conscientiously all safety equipment, devices, protective clothing and equipment that is fitted or made available. Wilful disregard of the Health and Safety at Work Act will lead to disciplinary action being taken under the practice's disciplinary procedure.

The practice will co-operate fully in the appointment of a safety representative and will provide him/her with sufficient facilities to carry out this task. The practice will also co-operate in the setting up of a safety committee should this be required.

Location

This policy applies to the premises of Ely Bridge Surgery and Cathedral Road Surgery.

Safety officer

The safety officer is ...., Practice Manager.

Safety representative

The safety representative is ...., Receptionist.

A safety representative is a person appointed from among the employees to speak for the employees in consultation with the practice and to undertake such other functions as may be prescribed. The practice has a duty to consult within these safety arrangements, which will enable us and our employees to co-operate in promoting and developing measures to ensure health and safety at work, and in checking the effectiveness of such measures.

The functions of the safety representative are:

* to represent the employees in consultation with the practice
* to investigate potential hazards and dangerous occurrences at the workplace and to examine the causes of accidents
* to investigate complaints by any employee he represents relating to that employee's health, safety, or welfare at work
* to carry out inspections
* to report the result of any inspection or investigation to the nominated safety officer.

Accidents

All accidents involving injury must:

* be reported to the reception supervisor and subsequently brought to the practice manager's attention

- be entered in the accident book by the injured person or nominee (giving all relevant details of place, people involved and account of how the accident happened). The accident book is kept near the switchboard at Ely Bridge Surgery.

First aid

There are two qualified first aiders, who are identified on the first aid notices in the reception area. First aid boxes are located behind the reception desk on the ground floor at Ely Bridge Surgery and in the records office in Cathedral Road Surgery.

Fire prevention

Fires always have a cause, therefore:

- smoking is not permitted on the premises
- switch machines off at night and remove plugs from sockets
- do not stand portable heaters where they can be knocked over
- do not place paper, towels, or clothing near portable fires
- never prop open a fire door.

Extreme care must be taken with storage and use of any flammable liquids.

- Do not use naked flames.
- Replace caps or stoppers of containers at once after use.
- Mop up any spillage and store mopping up material in a closed metal container before final disposal.

Fire precautions

You must make sure that you have read and understood the fire instructions that are to be found in each surgery.

- Find out the arrangements for the evacuation of the premises.
- Identify all exit routes, in case the normal one is blocked.

- When evacuating the surgery ensure that all windows and doors are closed behind you and that nobody remains behind.

If you have to pass through smoke to reach an escape route:

- inhale as little as possible
- keep near to the floor if the smoke is very dense.

If your route is impassable due to very dense smoke: close the door to your room and use the telephone to state your position

- make your presence known by standing at the window
- prevent smoke penetration around the door by sealing with whatever material you have available.

Bomb scares and other hazards

In the event of a bomb scare you should not close doors or windows. You should vacate the premises in accordance with instructions given by the practice manager or police.

Electrical equipment

You should look out for and report:

- loose connections
- non-earthed equipment
- damaged cables
- defective insulation
- overloaded circuits
- broken switches
- worn or dangerous appliances
- trailing leads
- liquids that if spilled could cause a short circuit.

All such hazards should be reported to the safety officer and the safety representative in writing. You should not attempt to repair or modify electrical equipment.

Office machinery and equipment

Paper cutting machines should be used on a stable surface and should never be left with the knife in the raised position.

Machines must only be operated by authorized users in accordance with the manufacturer's instructions. In the event of a failure, members of staff should not attempt to repair the machine unless authorized to do so, but should report the fault to the practice manager.

Electrically operated machines should only be operated with dry hands, and the supply should be switched off before maintenance is attempted by a person authorized to do so. Light and power cables should not be permitted to trail across floor space. Equipment should be positioned so that it does not create an obstacle for other staff.

Care should be taken to ensure that open drawers are closed after use, and only one drawer at a time should be opened to avoid the risk of the cabinet toppling. Personnel dealing with filing should take care to avoid cuts on fingers from paper edges and paper clips. Filing racks should be secured firmly to the adjacent wall or should be in a position where they cannot be pushed over.

Materials should be properly stored on racks, with heavy objects on the lower shelves. The shelves of storage racks should not be used as a means of access to the top shelves. When using a stepladder, care should be taken not to stand on tiptoe, to overreach, or to overbalance. A chair should not be used as a substitute for a stepladder.

Floor space

Many accidents at work are caused by falling. You should look out for the following and report them to the safety officer:

* missing or damaged handrails
* worn floor coverings
* wet/slippery floor surfaces
* broken glass
* trailing telephone or electric leads.

Obstructions should not be left in passageways. They may include:

- furniture
- cartons
- trolleys.

Escape routes must *never* be blocked.
Furniture can cause accidents, so you should remember not to:

- leave your desk drawer open
- put too much weight in the upper drawer of a filing cabinet
- open more than one filing cabinet drawer at a time
- position furniture where sharp corners could cause injury.

Lifting and carrying

Members of staff should not attempt to lift or move objects beyond their capabilities. When lifting a heavy package, staff should squat rather than stoop, keeping the weight close to the body and the back straight.

Computer equipment

Visual display units (VDUs) are used extensively in the practice. They have been blamed – often wrongly – for a wide range of health problems. In most areas the problems do not arise from the VDUs themselves, but from the way in which they are used.

You should ensure that the VDU is well positioned and that your work area is adequately lit. Any drifting, flickering, or jittering images should be reported so that any problems may be corrected.

If you experience aches or pains in the hands, wrists, arms, neck, or back (ie in the musculoskeletal system) after long periods of uninterrupted VDU work, you should alert the practice manager. Most problems of this type can be prevented by good workplace design and working practices.

As part of our commitment to a safe workplace, the practice will:

- analyse work-stations to assess and reduce risks
- ensure that work-stations meet minimum requirements

- on request, arrange an eyesight test for employees
- provide health and safety training
- provide information on health and safety matters.

Each employee should adjust his work-station to suit his requirements and avoid health problems, as follows.

- Adjust your chair and VDU to find the most comfortable position for your work. As a broad guide, your arms should be approximately horizontal and your eyes at the same height as the top of the VDU casing.

- Make sure there is enough space underneath your desk to move your legs freely. Move any obstacles such as boxes or equipment.

- Avoid excess pressure on the backs of your legs and knees. A foot rest, particularly for smaller users, may be helpful.

- Do not sit in the same position for long periods. Make sure you change your posture as often as practical. Some movement is desirable, but avoid repeated stretching movements.

- Adjust your keyboard and screen to get a good keying and viewing position. A space in front of the keyboard is sometimes helpful for resting the hands and wrists while not keying.

- Do not bend your hands up at the wrists when keying. Try to keep a soft touch on the keys and do not overstretch your fingers. Good keyboard technique is important.

- Try different layouts for keyboard, screen and document holder to find the best arrangement for you.

- Make sure you have enough work space to take whatever documents you need. A document holder may help you to avoid awkward neck movements.

- Arrange your desk and screen so that bright lights are not reflected in the screen. You should avoid directly facing windows or bright lights. Adjust curtains or blinds to prevent unwanted light.

- Make sure the characters on your screen are sharply focused and can be read easily. They should not flicker or move.

- Make sure there are no layers of dirt, grime, or finger marks on the screen.

- Use the brightness control on the screen to suit the lighting conditions in the room.

If you have problems that you think might be connected with your VDU work, you should talk to the practice manager, safety representative, or your own GP.

Guidance for staff involved in the handling of specimens of blood and body fluids

General precautions

Any cuts, grazes, or other forms of wound, particularly on the hands, must be covered by a waterproof dressing before you start work. The cover must be adequate to prevent contamination, and if you are not sure of the dressing's effectiveness you should ask the practice manager.

To help to protect both yourself and others with whom you come into contact:

- never take food, drink, cigarettes etc into any clinical area
- eating, drinking, chewing, smoking and applying cosmetics in the clinical areas are forbidden.

If you think that your hands or gloves may have been in direct contact with blood, body fluids, or other biological material:

- stop work at once
- discard the gloves, if wearing them
- wash your hands.

If a glove becomes perforated during work, even if you are not injured:

- stop work immediately
- remove the glove
- dispose of it into the appropriate bin
- wash your hands and put on a new glove.

If you have, or are involved in, an accidental breakage of equipment and/or spillage of material that could be infectious, you must report the incident at once. You must not attempt to do the decontamination yourself if you are not sure of the required techniques – you should ask a member of the nursing staff to deal with it. You should also make sure that any spilled materials are properly cleared away. Any broken equipment, particulary if the pieces could cause puncture wounds or cuts, must be placed in a container that provides protection for those who handle it. All used cleaning materials must be placed in an appropriate marked bin and disposed of appropriately.

Special work activities in the practice, eg disinfection, autoclaving and cleaning, must only be performed according to the written instructions. You should always follow these instructions – you must never change a procedure unless instructed to do so to meet special circumstances by the practice manager or other responsible person on the nursing staff.

If you are likely to be splashed by pathological materials, you must put on a fullface visor, gloves and a disposable plastic apron over your clothes.

If you become ill, you must remember to tell your doctor where you work. You should ask your doctor to talk to one of the medical staff in the practice if further information is required.

You should not take unnecessary risks and should always follow the above rules and those for your particular job category.

Precautions for staff involved in the taking of blood specimens

The work of phlebotomists/venepuncturists involves the collection of blood using aseptic techniques from patients whose history of infectivity may be unknown. Blood is collected by venepuncture or with a sterile disposable lancet. Staff will therefore be exposed to the risks associated with the constant handling of blood specimens in the presence of sharps. As well as following the general precautions outlined above, phlebotomists and venepuncturists must in addition observe the following points.

- Wear the gown or coverall provided for your protection.

- Wear gloves as required by practice rules and always when attending patients where a high risk of infection is suspected or known to exist.

- Do not take blood samples in offices or general work rooms in the practice. A consulting room must be set aside for taking blood specimens.

- Discard the gown/coverall worn during sampling immediately if it becomes contaminated with blood, and/or at the end of each day.

- Wash your hands between attending patients and at the end of each work period if they become contaminated. Cuts and grazes etc must be covered (see below).

- Do not deal with high-risk patients unless you have been specially trained. As well as wearing gloves, safety glasses or (preferably) a full-face visor should be worn according to medical advice.

- Remove needles from the syringe or other sampling device using forceps or another approved device. Needles must not be re-sheathed unless a safe procedure is available, in which case they should be disposed of without disassembly.

- After removing the needle from the syringe, transfer the blood carefully to avoid external contamination of the specimen container. Containers must be clearly labelled to indicate any known or suspected risk, and details provided on the accompanying paperwork. Care must be taken not to overpressurize the container.

- When using the 'vacutainer' method, reinsert the needle into the cover by use of the removal device provided. This will then allow safe removal of the covered needle from the vacutainer holder for disposal in the sharps box.

- Place specimen containers in a specimen transport bag before taking them from the bleeding site to laboratory collection point. Labels and paperwork must be checked for accuracy and the paperwork placed in the separate pocket of the transport bag.

- Dispose of syringes, needles and disposable lancets safely – directly into a sharps container and not into waste sacks.

- Clean the arm rest used for bleeding patients regularly using fresh disinfectant, preferably after each patient. Any spillage must be dealt with immediately.

Precautions for the handling of blood and other body fluid specimens by reception staff

Although the work of reception staff will involve handling bags and packages containing specimens to be sent to the laboratory for clinical examination, they are not required to come into direct contact with anything known to be infectious. Due to the possibility of accidentally doing so, however, they must always follow the general precautions given above as well as the guidelines specifically for staff in this work category.

- Never lick labels. Use either a roller pad or damp sponge or self-adhesive.

- Make sure that you clearly understand the hazard warning labels used on specimens.

- Wear gloves when instructed to do so by medical or nursing staff.

- If a leaking or broken specimen is found, do not touch it or any others on which it has leaked. Ask a member of the medical or nursing staff to deal with it if you have not received training in decontamination and cleaning techniques.

- Do not unpack or remove from its plastic bag any specimen with a label indicating a danger of infection. It must be delivered directly and unopened to the relevant laboratory.

- Keep all specimens together in the collection box. Never put them on a desk or elsewhere where a leak could cause a direct risk to yourself or those with whom you work.

- Twice each day, eg before lunch and when you finish work for the day, the specimen collection box should be washed down thoroughly with freshly prepared disinfectant using disposable cloths or paper towels. Dispose of the cleaning cloths safely.

- Wash your hands frequently during the course of your daily work – always before a break and at the end of the day. Wash them at once if they become contaminated by a specimen.

Accidental injury involving specimens or sharps

In the event of a needlestick or sharps injury involving blood or body fluids, the following steps should be taken.

- Encourage bleeding and wash liberally with soap and water.

- Report all such incidents to the reception supervisor/practice manager.

- Ascertain the details of the incident and ensure that they are recorded in the accident book. Important details include:

  —time of the incident
  —type of incident
  —source of the needle/sharp instrument
  —whether the donor can be identified
  —whether the donor is in an identified high-risk group
  —whether the staff member has received hepatitis B immunization.

- Contact one of the partners who will advise appropriate action and may arrange for blood testing.

Guidance for cleaning staff in clinical areas

The work of cleaning staff, including contractors, may involve accidental contact with materials that could be infectious. As well as the general precautions outlined above, cleaning staff must also observe the following safe working practices.

- Always wear the overall provided for your protection when working in clinical areas and see that it is properly fastened.

- Wash your hands often while at work, particularly after you have handled clinical equipment.

- Cover cuts and grazes with waterproof dressings so that materials in clinical areas cannot get into them. You may sometimes be instructed to wear gloves.

- If you have an accident of any kind, or knock over any bottle, jar or tube, or piece of equipment, tell your supervisor or one of the nursing staff at once. Make sure that the matter is reported because the accident may have caused infectious material to be spilled.

- Do not place broken glass in plastic disposal bags; use the labelled sharps containers provided for this purpose.

- When handling dirty glassware, wear heavy-duty gloves. Be very careful when putting your hands into bowls or other receptacles which may contain glassware items, as some could be broken and could cause cuts.

Guidance for staff operating the autoclave

- Do not attempt to use the autoclave until you have been taught how to do so and the responsible member of the nursing staff is satisfied that you are competent.

- Follow the operating instructions displayed near to the autoclave at all times.

- Do not allow items requiring autoclaving to accumulate. They will be infectious and the risks are likely to get worse if not dealt with straight away.

- If you have to stack waste containers or other materials awaiting autoclaving, do so carefully. If stacks collapse or fall over, the spilt material could spread infection. If waste or other materials are spilled, report it to the safety officer at once and get instructions on how to deal with it. Do not try to do it yourself if you have not been trained to decontaminate spillage.

- If the pressure or temperature indication is incorrect, report it. Do not use the autoclave if you suspect that it is not working properly. If there are any doubts, all the material already in the chamber must be autoclaved again.

Guidance for staff involved in the handling of clinical waste

- When collecting waste from disposal points, make sure that it is properly bagged or otherwise safely contained.

- Some sharps containers may leak and sharp objects can be pushed through the sides. Be very careful when handling them because both the liquids and the sharp points can cause infection. Always wear heavy-duty gloves. If any of the liquid spills on your overall you must change it. If any gets on your gloves, wash them at once.

- Always use the specially provided waste sacks and ensure that these are safely stored in the locked clinical waste container.

Staff handbook – an example

Foreword

The aim of this handbook is to help you. It provides clear information on aspects of your conditions of service and highlights some of your obligations to the practice. All that is included stems from your contract of employment with the practice, which is based on current legislation. If you have any questions or concerns please speak to the practice manager or staff partner. Part of their job is to make you feel happy and content at the practice. This practice is a leader in the NHS in South Glamorgan because we work as a team and we work hard. To achieve this we are always concerned that members of staff get job satisfaction and know they are valued.

Welcome to the team.

Disclaimer

Any reference in these documents to employees being male is used simply as a means of illustration. It is intended that the documents will be applied equally to all male and female employees.

This copy issued to: .... (name)

on: .... (date)

Introduction

The purpose of this handbook is to welcome all staff to the Ely Bridge Practice and to provide you with information to help you settle into your new job. It also provides staff in post with up-to-date information on their employment.

Written particulars of employment

On appointment you will be given two copies of the *Terms and conditions of employment* of your post. You should sign one copy and return it to the practice manager. The second copy is for your retention. Once you are in post, you will receive a copy of any amendment reflecting any changes to your contract. This normally happens in May each year.

Hours of work

The normal hours of work are between 8.30 am and 6.30 pm Monday to Friday depending on the shift pattern. Many staff work flexible hours, however, to meet the demands of the service. This includes Saturday mornings.

Conditions of service

The main details will be stated in your contract of employment. You will be paid monthly, normally on the 28th day of each month. Your monthly salary is calculated as 1/12th of your annual salary. Salaries are paid by direct transfer to your bank or building society account. A payslip will be given to you at the end of the month, on which your gross pay and various deductions will be noted. You are advised to keep your monthly payslips (and form P60 which is issued to you every April) for tax and benefit purposes.

Income tax

If this is your first job on leaving school you will need to complete form P46 so that you can be given your correct tax code. If this is not your first job, on your first day you should, if possible, have with you your income tax form P45, which will be needed by the payroll officer to ensure that the correct amount of tax is deducted from your pay.

National insurance

On your first day you should also have with you evidence of your national insurance number (obtainable from the DSS). Compulsory national insurance deductions will be made from your pay.

Birth certificate

On your first day you should bring with you your birth certificate so that your date of birth may be verified.

Change of personal circumstances

Please inform the practice manager in writing of any changes in your personal circumstances, eg change of name on marriage, change of address etc, so that accurate records may be maintained.

Sickness

A sick pay scheme, in accordance with existing agreements, is in operation. If you are unable to attend work because of illness, you or someone on your behalf must notify the practice manager as soon as possible, no later than 10.00 am on the first day of absence.

On return to work you are required to complete a self-certification form for absence from 4 to 7 days. For a period of absence of more than 7 days you are required to submit a medical certificate to the practice manager.

In certain circumstances you may be required to undergo an independent medical examination. You should, where possible, inform the practice manager in advance of the date of your return to work following absence on sick leave.

If your absence on account of sickness is due to active participation in sport as a profession or arises from or is attributable to your own misconduct, you have no automatic right to sick pay. Further details may be obtained from the practice manager.

Notice is taken of sickness statistics and in cases of regular sickness an informal interview may be arranged.

Welfare

If you have a problem at home or in the office (which is affecting your work) the staff partner may be able to help you. Your business will be confidential unless you give permission for it to be discussed.

Accidents

If you are involved in an accident at work, you must report the matter to the practice manager and ensure that full details of the accident are entered in the accident book, which is retained by the switchboard in the Records Room.

First aid

The names of qualified first aiders are listed on the relevant signs. There is first aid and emergency resuscitation equipment located at the main reception desk in both the main and branch surgeries. In the case of a serious accident, please dial 999 for an ambulance which will take the injured person to Cardiff Royal Infirmary.

Health and Safety at Work Act 1974

The Act that came into force on 1 April 1975 was introduced to protect all employees from risks that may arise at work. The Act provided that it shall be the duty of every employee while at work to take reasonable care for the health and safety of himself and of other persons who may be affected by his actions. The practice also has a responsibility to ensure a healthy working environment and safe working systems. Please refer to the separate booklet outlining the practice health and safety policy.

Any possible safety hazard should be immediately referred to the practice manager.

Fire

You must read and understand the fire instructions which are strategically placed throughout the building. If you discover a fire, you should sound the nearest fire alarm button (located near the front door and rear entrances on the ground floor and in the central lobby on the first floor).

Your may attack the fire with an extinguisher if it is felt safe to do so. Please remember:

- black carbon dioxide (CO_2) extinguisher – for use on electrical fires and burning liquids only
- red water extinguisher – all other fires.

On hearing the fire alarm you should lock away any confidential documents and shut all doors and windows. You must not stop to collect personal belongings. You should leave the building by the nearest exit and assemble at the far side of the car park.

All staff will check their own area. The fire officer, who is the senior member of the partnership present, will make a final check of the building. It will be the responsibility of the fire officer to summon the fire and rescue services, if necessary.

You must not return to the building until all personnel are accounted for and you are told it is safe to do so by the fire officer.

Flexi hours

A system of flexi hours is in operation for all staff. When you work in excess of your contracted hours, you may take this time as flexi leave, subject to the exigencies of the service. In this way a flexi leave balance can be built up. This should not exceed 3 working days (pro rata) in value.

Any flexi leave earned or taken must be recorded on the appropriate form held by the practice manager. Management does not encourage the taking of accumulated flexi leave in less than half day units.

Standards of appearance

All members of staff are required to conform to standards of dress and appearance appropriate to their employment, particularly as most staff are in regular contact with members of the public.

Male members of staff are expected to be clean shaven (unless purposely bearded), and it is suggested a tie is worn under normal weather conditions.

Trades union

You are entitled to join a trades union. Deduction of trades union subscriptions from your pay can be arranged with your approval.

Leave

Leave (general)

Leave is to be arranged in consultation with the practice manager and the appropriate form is to be completed before leave is taken.

Hospital and dental appointments

Staff are expected to arrange non-urgent hospital, medical, or dental appointment in their own time or to adjust their working hours accordingly. Only under exceptional circumstances will paid time off be permitted. All requests for time off should be directed to the practice manager.

Annual leave

Your entitlement for this and subsequent years is shown on your written statement of *Main Terms and Conditions of Employment* – for the majority of staff this will be 25 days a year (pro rata for part-time staff). The leave year for all staff runs from 1 April to 31 March.

Staff are required to forecast their leave requirements for the summer period at least 3 months in advance; 4 weeks notice is required for other periods of annual leave (ie 4 days or more). No particular dates can be guaranteed until the leave sheet is signed, and the staffing requirement of the practice will take precedence.

Unpaid leave

There is no entitlement to unpaid leave. In exceptional circumstances an application will be considered on its merit. Such an application should be made in writing to the practice manager.

Compassionate leave

Compassionate leave may be granted to a member of staff in appropriate circumstances. A letter of application should be given to the practice manager. Each case will be judged on its merit. In urgent cases the practice manager should be telephoned for approval.

Special leave

Full details of special leave that may be granted, (eg for training with the Reserve and Cadet Forces) are available from the practice manager.

Study leave

If you wish to apply for study leave to undertake further training appropriate to your present or future employment within the health service you should consult the staff partner as soon as possible. When granting study leave, consideration will be given to the number of staff away from the practice at any one time. All staff are encouraged to undertake further training applicable to their work.

Maternity leave

Full-time (and some part-time) female staff with a minimum of 26 weeks service may be entitled to maternity benefit. The amount of benefits dependent on the length of service and may include:

- paid maternity leave of up to 18 weeks
- unpaid maternity leave for up to 22 weeks from the end of the paid period of leave. If you should fail to return to work with this practice following notification of your intention to do so, you will be liable to refund all of the maternity pay received except for the 6 weeks' pay entitlement.

Exact details may be obtained from the practice manager, as legislation and FHSA guidance changes from time to time. You should ask for the latest information.

Overtime

Overtime is only worked with the prior approval of the practice manager. Overtime is not payable until a total of 37.5 hours (or pro rata equivalent) has been worked within the current working week. Overtime is only payable for completed half hours.

Members of staff are contracted to work compulsory overtime should this ever be necessary. Normally 48 hours' notice would be given.

Resignation

If you decide to leave your employment you should give notice by formal letter to the practice manager in accordance with the terms of your contract for employment. Shortly after termination, your final pay and form P45 (which shows details of your pay to date since 6 April and the income tax deducted) will be forwarded to you. If you are going to further employment, your new employer will need your P45 to ensure that the correct deductions are made from your pay.

Training

Most staff are required to undergo training soon after arrival which will assist them in their particular work. A variety of courses is available, and the staff partner may be contacted for details.

While there will obviously be no compulsion to attend training courses, it should be realized that staff members who do undergo training place themselves in a better position for promotion when opportunities occur. Given equal performance, a trained person will obviously be preferred to an untrained one, regardless of seniority in post.

Staff intending to make a career in the health service will be expected to attend a suitable training course.

Confidentiality

Matters of a confidential nature with which your work brings you into contact, both clinical and commercial, must not be discussed with any unauthorized person. Disciplinary action will be taken against any employee responsible for a breach of confidentiality. In serious cases this may mean instant dismissal.

Loss of personal effects

The practice does not accept liability for any loss of personal property from any part of the premises, with the exception of small items of value handed to the practice manager for safe custody and for which a receipt has been issued. Members of staff are requested not to bring items of value or significant sums of money into the office.

Compensation will be considered for damage to clothing occurring during the course of a task, but staff are expected to act reasonably.

Use of equipment and materials

You are responsible for any practice equipment in your charge and for putting away any attractive, transportable items at the end of work each day.

Extreme weather conditions

Persons living over 1 mile away from the practice, provided that public transport is not running, would not be expected to report to the practice but could stay at home and consideration would be given to full payment of salary due.

Annual appraisals

All staff will be subject to an annual appraisal. Details of the procedure are available from the staff partner.

Disciplinary and grievance procedures

Purpose and scope

The practice expects its staff to observe a high standard of conduct, attendance and job performance. The disciplinary rules that apply to you in your employment can also be found in your contract of employment. The disciplinary procedure sets out what action will be taken when these rules are breached.

Principles

- No disciplinary action will be taken until a case has been fully investigated. This will, wherever possible, be undertaken by an independent third party to the issue.

- At every stage in the procedures you will be given the opportunity to state your case and to be accompanied by a colleague at any formal interview.

- The investigation does not form part of any disciplinary procedure. To facilitate a prompt and impartial investigation, you may be suspended on full pay while the investigation takes place.

- You will have the right to appeal to the staff partner against any disciplinary penalty (*see later under* Appeals).

Procedures

Stage 1: Verbal warning

If your conduct or performance is unsatisfactory, you will normally be given warning which will be recorded. The warning will state the nature of the misconduct, your right to appeal and the period of time given for improvement.

Stage 2: Written warning

If the offence is serious or if there is continued cause for concern after a verbal warning, a written warning will be given stating the nature of complaint, the improvement required and the timescale. You will be advised of your right of appeal and that if there is no satisfactory improvement, a final warning will be given. A copy of this written warning will be kept but it will be discharged after 6 months subject to satisfactory conduct and performance.

Stage 3: Final written warning

If conduct or performance is still unsatisfactory after a first written warning or if the offence is of a more serious nature, a final written warning will be given stating the nature of the complaint and that dismissal will result if there is no satisfactory improvement. You will be advised of the right of appeal. A copy of the final written warning will be kept but it will be discharged after 6 months subject to satisfactory conduct and performance.

Stage 4: Dismissal

If there is no satisfactory improvement or if you commit a more serious offence, dismissal will normally result. You will be given the reason for dismissal, the termination date and the right of appeal.

Gross misconduct

In the case of gross misconduct it may be appropriate to dismiss you without regard to stages 1–3. Examples of gross misconduct include theft, breach of confidentiality and assault. In certain circumstances, the procedure to be followed may involve immediate suspension from duty on full pay so that enquiries may be made. If the allegations are confirmed after the investigation and after your response, if any, the result will be summary dismissal.

Appeals

If you are dissatisfied with any disciplinary decision that affects you, you should appeal in writing within 2 working days to the staff partner whose decision will be final.

Grievances

If you should have a grievance about your employment you should apply in the first instance to the practice manger. You should explain your grievance verbally in the first instance. If you are not satisfied with the response, you should put your grievance in writing and forward it to the staff partner.

K   Assistance with business planning

This book has, we hope, convinced you of the need for effective business planning in your practice. However, where do you turn for help?

The Department for Enterprise (formerly the DTI) has a Business Planning Initiative which allows for a sliding scale of reimbursement against the costs of consultancy advice. You will have to pay two thirds of the cost agreed between you and the consultant. If you are located in an Assisted Area or Urban Programme Area, you will only have to pay half the agreed consultancy cost. It should be noted that the reimbursement is only possible if you use your own, that is not NHS, funds.

However, this would apparently not prohibit the costs being charged in full to the preparatory year fee or management allowance for fundholding practices, subject to FHSA approval.

Effective business planning typically requires from five to 15 days of consultancy, with daily rates for consultants varying from £250 to £500. Again, these charges depend on your location and the regional offices of the Department of Enterprise can provide further details.

You may now be confident enough to draft your own business plan. The 'number crunching' could be delegated to your practice accountant who will have the dual advantage of being familiar with your affairs, and cost less than a management consultant!

Regional offices of the Department of Enterprise

DTI North East
Cleveland, Durham, Northumberland and Tyne & Wear

Stanegate House, 2 Groat Market, Newcastle-upon-Tyne, NE1 1YN
Telephone: 091-235 7292, Telex: 53178 DOITYNG
Fax: 091-232 6742

DTI North West (Manchester)

Cheshire (except Chester, Widnes/Runcorn), Cumbria, Lancashire, Greater Manchester and the High Peak District of Derbyshire

Sunley Tower, Piccadilly Plaza, Manchester M1 4BA
Telephone: 061-838 5000, Telex: 666382 DTINWM,
Fax: 061-838 5236

DTI Yorkshire and Humberside

North Yorkshire, South Yorkshire, West Yorkshire and Humberside

25 Queen Street, Leeds LS1 2TW, Telephone: (0532) 338300,
Telex: 557925 DTILDSG, Fax: (0532) 338301/2

DTI East Midlands

Nottinghamshire, Derbyshire (except the High Peak District), Leicestershire, Lincolnshire and Northamptonshire

Severns House, 20 Middle Pavement, Nottingham NG1 7DW
Telephone: (0602) 596460, Telex: 37143 DTINOTG
Fax: (0602) 587074

DTI West Midlands

The Metropolitan districts of Birmingham, Coventry, Dudley, Sandwell, Solihull, Walsall and Wolverhampton, and the counties of Warwickshire, Shropshire, Staffordshire and Hereford & Worcester

77 Paradise Circus, Queensway, Birmingham B1 2DT
Telephone: 021-212 5000, Telex: 337919 DTIBHMG
Fax: 021-212 1010

DTI East

Bedfordshire, Cambridgeshire, Essex, Hertfordshire, Norfolk and Suffolk,

The Westbrook Centre, Milton Road, Cambridge CB4 1YG
Telephone: (0223) 461939, Telex: 81582 DTIEAO
Fax: (0223) 461941

DTI South East London

Greater London

Bridge Place, 88–89 Eccleston Square, London SW1V 1PT
Telephone: 071-627 7800, Telex: 297124 SEREXG, Fax: 071-828 1105

DTI South East (Reading)
Berkshire, Buckinghamshire, Hampshire, Oxfordshire and Isle of Wight

40 Caversham Road, Reading RG1 7EB, Telephone: (0734) 395600,
Telex: 847799 DTIRDG, Fax: (0734) 502818

DTI South East (Reigate)
Kent, Surrey (outside Greater London boundary),
East Sussex and West Sussex

Douglas House, London Road, Reigate RH2 9QP
Telephone: (0737) 226900, Telex: 918364 DTIRGTG
Fax: (0737) 223491

DTI South West
Avon, Cornwall (including Scilly Isles), Devon, Dorset, Gloucestershire,
Somerset and Wiltshire

The Pithay, Bristol BS1 2PB, Telephone: (0272) 308400
Telex: 44214 DTIBTLG, Fax: (0272) 299494

Scotland
Enterprise Services, Scotland Ltd, Apex 1, 99 Haymarket Terrace,
Edinburgh EH12 5HD, Telephone: 031-313 6200, Fax: 031-313 2378

for other Enterprise Initiative enquiries contact:

The Scottish Office, Industry Department, Alhambra House,
45 Waterloo Street, Glasgow G2 6AT
Telephone: 041-248 4774 (24 hour answering service)

Wales
North and South Wales
Clwyd, Dyfed (except the Ceredigion District),
Gwynedd (except the Meirionnydd District), West Glamorgan,
Mid Glamorgan, South Glamorgan and Gwent

Welsh Development Agency, Enterprise Initiative Unit,
Business Development Centre, Treforest Industrial Estate,
Mid Glamorgan CF37 5UR
Telephone: (0443) 841200 (24 hour answering service)
Fax: (0443) 841121

Mid Wales
Powys, the Meirionnydd District of Gwynedd and the
Ceredigion District of Dyfed

Development Board for Rural Wales, Ladywell House, Newtown,
Mid Wales SY16 1JB, Dial 100 and ask for Freephone New Wales
Fax: (0686) 622 499

for other Enterprise Initiative enquiries contact:

The Welsh Office Industry Department, New Crown Buildings,
Cathays Park, Cardiff CF1 3NQ
Telephone: (0222) 823185 (24 hour answering service)

Index